MEDICARE MADE SIMPLE

A CONSUMER'S GUIDE TO THE MEDICARE PROGRAM

Denise Knaus

Library of Congress Cataloging-in-Publication Data

Knaus, Denise L.
    Medicare made simple / Denise Knaus.
        p.   cm.
    Includes bibliographical references.
    ISBN 1-885987-00-5
    1. Medicare--Handbooks, manuals, etc.
    2. Medicare--Dictionaries.
    I. Title.
    HD7102.U4K63   1996
    344.73'0226--dc20
    [347.304226]   96-11124
                                                                  CIP

ISBN: 1-885987-00-5

Printed in the United States of America

Health Information Press
4727 Wilshire Blvd., Suite 300
Los Angeles, CA 90010
1-800-MED-SHOP
email: MEDICALBOOKSTORE.COM

ABOUT THE AUTHOR

Denise Knaus is president and owner of Knaus and Associates, a practice management, reimbursement and Medicare consulting firm in the Chicago area. In addition, she teaches workshops on coding, reimbursement and Medicare regulations for physician practices, clinics, hospitals and medical associations, including the American Academy of Family Physicians.

Knaus regularly contributes articles to industry newsletters on the subject of Medicare regulations. She has authored workbooks on Medicare, as well as coding and reimbursement, including *The Biller's Guide to Insurance* published by the American Medical Association, and *Medicare Rules and Regulations*, published by Practice Management Information Corp. (PMIC).

Knaus received her BBA degree from the University of Iowa.

DISCLAIMER

This publication is designed to offer basic and practical information on Medicare. The information presented is based on the experience and interpretation of the author. Although the information has been carefully researched and checked for accuracy, currency and completeness, neither the author nor the publisher accept any responsibility or liability with regard to errors, omissions, misuse or misinterpretation.

CONTENTS

FOREWORD

When the Medicare program was enacted in 1965, it was intended to help improve access to health care for the elderly by offsetting some of the costs associated with medical care. Thirty years later, this is still the basic intent of the program. However, whether the program achieves this goal has come under greater public scrutiny and public and congressional debate.

Do the "beneficiaries" actually "benefit" from this program? Or has it become so complicated—with its myriad rules and regulations governing everything from what is covered to how to complete a form—that the beneficiaries are actually being caused more harm from the stress of understanding their benefits than the benefits actually provide?

It is with these questions in mind that this book was written. After enjoying success with a publication designed to help physician practices understand and adhere to Medicare regulations, I felt the time had come to create a hands-on, practical, and accurate publication designed for those people who are actually *using* the benefits provided by the Medicare program.

My goal is to provide practical and easy-to-understand information about the Medicare program and its benefits to those people it is supposed to "benefit." This book should help you understand the program so that you can obtain all the benefits to which you are entitled under Medicare.

Please note that it is not the intent of this book to "take a stand" or a political position on issues related to Medicare. The debate regarding coverage and cost of services provided to Medicare beneficiaries is better left to the beneficiary population and their representatives in Congress. This book is intended to help you understand the program and its workings so you can better utilize your benefits—and encounter less stress in the process.

This book focuses on Medicare and those issues concerning Medicare entitlement, enrollment, coverage of services, payment methods and requirements, alternatives to traditional fee-for-service care, appeals, and fraud and abuse, to name a few. The Social Security Administration (SSA), the Health Care Financing Administration (HCFA), and other government agencies have published pamphlets on different Medicare topics. However, these publications provide neither depth nor breadth in their coverage of the subject. They usually address only one topic, such as coverage or enrollment, and don't provide practical help in solving problems related to your coverage or other issues.

If you feel that an issue is not discussed, or not in enough depth, or if you would like to see additional topics added to this book, please write to the author in care of the publisher. It is our goal to provide a complete, up-to-date, and practical guide that will help you understand your Medicare benefits and get the most from them. Direct your comments to:

Denise Knaus, Author
Medicare Made Simple
c/o Health Information Press
4727 Wilshire Boulevard, Suite 300
Los Angeles, CA 90010
(213) 954-0224

For ease in reading, the generic pronoun "he" has been used in place of "he/she." No discrimination is intended.

All deductible and coinsurance dollar amounts are for calendar year 1996. Please contact your local Social Security office or Medicare carrier for other figures.

ACKNOWLEDGMENTS

Many people deserve acknowledgment for their assistance with this book:

Thank you to Charles Owen in HCFA's Bureau of Data Management and Strategy, Office of Statistics and Data Management, who provided claims and expenditure statistics, and to George Lintzeris in HCFA's Bureau of Data Management and Strategy, Office of Health Care Information Systems, who assisted with expenditure statistics.

Thanks to the Downers Grove, Illinois, Social Security Administration Office for help in understanding the process of Social Security enrollment and Medicare enrollment.

Kathy Canney of PSC in Lombard, Illinois, was a great help in providing contacts for Part A information.

Legal Counsel for the Elderly provided invaluable information for Chapter Seven, for which I am grateful.

Thank you to Corinne Brophy, Cynthia Knaus, Laura Tatten, Barbara Martin, Mary Alice Kill, Bob and Ethel Yarbro, Rex and Esther Yarbro, Gloria Wanland, Delman Campbell, Anna Lopuh, Cathy Epstein, and George Walker for their contributions to my beneficiary survey. And thanks to William Yarbro and Ray McGinness for their help with the Medicare Benefit Notices for Part A Services.

Much gratitude is due Carol Smith Pynchon, who worked tirelessly to edit this book. It is her talents that organized some of the chapters, made some very technical information easier to understand, and completed not-so-complete explanations.

Thank you to William Lessard for his knowledge and expertise in scrutinizing the book for factual accuracy.

Finally, thank you to my husband, Gary, for his support and help while I was working on this book, and to my beautiful daughters, Kaitlin and Claire, because they inspire me every day to be the best I can be.

Denise L. Knaus

INTRODUCTION

In my ten-plus years in the health care field, I have learned more than I ever wanted to know about the Medicare program. In that learning process, I have often felt that the very people intended to benefit from the Medicare program—the "beneficiaries"—are the same people who least understand it and experience the greatest amount of confusion and aggravation when trying to use their "benefits."

If you are one of these people, this book is for you. It is intended to help you understand your Medicare benefits and to give you guidance on how to cope with common issues and problems.

In discussions with Medicare beneficiaries and their families, these are some of the more common questions asked:

- How do I sign up for Medicare?

- How much does Medicare cost?

- What is supplemental insurance and how do I get it?

- What is a participating physician?

- Can I have HMO *and* Medicare?

- Who pays if I have Medicare and I have insurance from my spouse's employer?

- What do I do if Medicare doesn't pay for some services?

- Does it mean my doctor is a bad doctor if services he provides are denied as "not reasonable and necessary"?

- Should I send in a claim in addition to the claim my doctor sends in if Medicare is taking a long time to pay?

- Will Medicare pay for an annual physical exam?

- How do I know if my doctor is charging the right amount?

- Why am I getting a bill from the hospital? I thought Medicare would pay.

- Does Medicare pay for wheelchairs or nursing home care?

- What do I do if my doctor charges me for something he didn't do?

PURPOSE AND CONTENT

This book is designed as a reference guide to provide answers to such typical questions asked by Medicare beneficiaries and their families and representatives. Consider this book to be your professional "Medicare advisor." Just as you need accountants and lawyers to help with your taxes and legal issues, so you need an advisor to help you understand and work with the Medicare program.

Included in this introduction is a *brief* overview of the evolution of the Medicare program. This information should provide some perspective of the growth of the program, and shed some light on some of the reasons for Congressional attention to controlling Medicare expenditures.

Following this brief history, a "Glossary of Insurance Terminology" provides definitions of common insurance terms in plain, simple English. Once you are familiar with the terms, you will understand the contents of this book more readily. More importantly, you'll know the "jargon" so you can deal on a more equal level with physicians,✔ hospitals, and Medicare carriers and intermediaries.

Checklists and other practical tools are used throughout this guide. Where appropriate, step-by-step advice and guidance are provided to help you work through Medicare decisions and deal effectively with providers (hospitals, physicians, and suppliers) and Medicare contractors (carriers and intermediaries).

You will find information related to many topics, including:

- Determining your eligibility for Medicare benefits.

- Signing up for benefits.

- How to pay for your benefits.

- What services Medicare pays for and what services it does not.

- What types of practitioners can provide services under the Medicare program.

- How Medicare pays for services; when and how much you are responsible for paying.

- Making the decision regarding a supplemental policy or managed care plan.

- Activities that are considered fraud and abuse of the program.

- When another insurer should pay before Medicare pays.

Please note that this guide discusses *Medicare*. It provides information related to Social Security benefits only as it relates to Medicare eligibility. This book provides no information related to Medicaid.

Be aware that Medicare and Medicaid are separate and distinct programs serving different populations. While both are administered by the Health Care Financing Administration (HCFA), an agency of the Department of Health and Human Services, they are not intended for the same group of people. Medicare is available to persons aged 65 and over, disabled individuals, and people with end stage renal disease (kidney failure). Medicaid, on the other hand, is a program of medical benefits for the poor and indigent.

The Medicaid program is paid for by federal and state funds. Each state is responsible for administering its program, including making eligibility and coverage decisions, following federal guidelines. While Medicare beneficiaries can also receive Medicaid benefits, Medicaid recipients are not necessarily eligible for Medicare. If you are low-income or indigent, check with your local Social Security office or state welfare agency for additional information regarding eligibility for Medicaid benefits in your state.

EVOLUTION OF THE MEDICARE PROGRAM

The Medicare program was enacted by Congress in August 1965 as part of President Lyndon Johnson's "Great Society." President Johnson believed that in a land as prosperous as ours, we could afford to take care of everyone; no one should be left out of the great wealth. He spoke of the "Great Society" in his inaugural speech:

> *In a land of great wealth, families must not live in hopeless poverty. In a land rich in harvest, children must not go hungry. In a land of healing miracles, neighbors must not suffer and die unattended. In a land of great learning and scholars, young people must be taught to read and write.*

Medicare was designed to cover some of the cost of health care services to ensure access to a basic level of health care for the aged. Called the Health Insurance for the Aged and Disabled Act and passed as Title XVIII of the Social Security Act (which was passed in 1935), Medicare's specific purpose was to provide hospital and medical insurance benefits to the elderly (over age 65). Medicare began paying benefits in July 1966.

In the beginning, the Health Insurance for the Aged and Disabled Act provided insurance for inpatient hospital care, other inpatient care such as skilled nursing facilities, and home health care. This part of the law, officially titled "Hospital Insurance for the Aged and Disabled," is also known as "basic Medicare" or "Medicare Part A" because it's found in Part A of Title XVIII of the Social Security Act.

The Act also provided a supplementary program that covered the costs of physicians' services and other items and services not covered under Part A. Contained in Part B of Title XVIII of the Social Security Act, this program is officially titled "Supplementary Medical Insurance Benefits for the Aged and Disabled," but is often referred to as "Medicare Part B" or the "Supplementary Medical Insurance (SMI) Program."

The Hospital Insurance program (Part A) is funded by payroll taxes (listed as FICA on your pay stub) paid by individuals and their employers. Individuals are required to pay 1.45 percent of their earnings toward this insurance, with a matching amount paid by employers. Self-employed persons pay 2.9 percent for Hospital Insurance, but are allowed to deduct one-half of this amount on their income tax returns.

Medicare Part A is funded by FICA taxes. Part B insurance is funded by premiums collected from beneficiaries and by the federal government's general fund (primarily income taxes). Currently, premiums cover only one-fourth of the cost of the Part B program; the remainder is shouldered by the federal budget.

Benefits were initially available to persons 65 years of age and over. In 1972, amendments to the Act extended benefits to persons receiving Social Security disability benefits for more than two years, regardless of their age. Later, benefits were also extended to individuals who suffer from end stage renal disease (ESRD) regardless of their age, and to federal, state, and local government employees 65 years of age and older.

In addition to the expansion of those eligible for Medicare benefits, legislation has guaranteed coverage of some of the services provided by practitioners other than physicians. This includes physician assistants, nurse practitioners, chiropractors, podiatrists, and optometrists (see Chapter Three for specific services covered). Legislation has also expanded coverage for additional services, such as screening mammographies and durable medical equipment.

THE PROGRAM TODAY

Without presenting myriad statistics and embarking on long-winded economic and political discussions about the growth of the Medicare program, this section provides a *brief* explanation of the program's expansion and development.

It is important to realize that when the Medicare program began, it covered fewer people and fewer services than it does today. As the program expanded and more and more beneficiaries were added, a larger work force was needed to handle the increasing workload.

Remember that not only did legislation expand the beneficiary coverage, but also the elderly population as a whole grew over 60 percent. Thus, persons enrolled for Medicare coverage increased from 19.1 million in 1966 to 36.7 million in 1994—a 92 percent increase. This population growth increased the number of people who obtained coverage and submitted claims.

The Medicare program (both Parts A and B) processed an average of almost 1.5 claims per beneficiary in 1967; in 1994, this average had risen to 20.1 claims per beneficiary. In dollars, this translates to $4,741.14 spent per beneficiary in 1994 as compared to $167.54 in 1967.

In addition, special interest groups have influenced Congress to pass laws to protect beneficiaries. Some of these include the refund requirement for medically unnecessary services and providing advance notice for elective surgery costing over $500. These additional laws led to more and more rules and regulations, which in turn increased the program's administrative costs, not only to the government but also to the private sector, including hospitals, physicians, and other suppliers. Meanwhile, the beneficiaries' confusion and misunderstanding have grown as well.

Human Nature as a Factor

In addition to legislative changes, the framers of the original Act did not anticipate the possibility of a "blank check" mentality where, because a third party is paying the bill, charges increase at a rate greater than would be dictated by other economic factors. The number and types of services that are provided increase, sometimes without regard to the real necessity of the service.

Also, users of health care seek services more freely, and will seek more services, because someone else is paying the bill. All of these factors combined to produce an extremely large, unwieldy, and complicated program, both to understand and to administer.

The Medicare program began draining more and more dollars from the strained federal budget. Today, Medicare covers approximately 37.5 million beneficiaries and consumes approximately $159 billion—or 11.2 percent—of our federal budget. Of this total, $102 billion is expended for hospital services and $57 billion is spent on physician and other services.

The Congress (and many other people and sectors of our society) are very concerned about the growth of expenditures for health care, and most especially Medicare expenditures. This has caused Congress and its agencies to institute tighter controls on coverage, eligibility, and payments for services rendered. The focus is now on cost containment, for both the government and the beneficiaries.

While this explanation provides only a very cursory overview of factors affecting the growth of the program, it does help point out why the program has become so confusing and complex. The focus on cost containment has caused Medicare to be more sensitive to *what* is paid for and *when* it is paid. This translates to a concern about the medical necessity of the procedure and specifics regarding coverage of certain procedures and services. The more specific these guidelines and rules become, the more onerous they are to maintain, enforce, and administer.

GLOSSARY

Understanding health insurance and Medicare policies and procedures requires a fundamental working knowledge of the words and acronyms used by medical professionals, government agencies, and insurance carriers to describe services, benefits, and payment policies. While many publications place the terminology section in an appendix at the back of the book, I feel you should have an opportunity to review and learn the terminology *before* you encounter it within the text itself.

Abuse: Incidents or practices of physicians or other providers that, although not usually considered fraudulent, are inconsistent with accepted sound medical, business, or fiscal practice.

Accident Insurance: Insurance under which benefits are payable in case of accidental injury or accidental death.

Actual Charge: The amount that is billed or submitted for a service or procedure. The actual charge is one of the factors used to determine Medicare's payment and to establishing the customary, prevailing and reasonable (CPR) payment. *See also Fee Schedule; Customary, Prevailing and Reasonable.*

Adjudication: The claims processing cycle.

Administrative Law Judge (ALJ): A hearing official assigned to the Medicare Office of Hearings and Appeals.

Allowable Charge: The payment amount established by Medicare for a given procedure, service, or supply. This amount includes the payment from Medicare and the beneficiary's coinsurance amount, but does not include any balance bill amount. (*Note*: In this book, allowable is used to refer to the payment amount as it is determined by Medicare.) *Also called* Approved Charge. *See also Balance Bill; Coinsurance; Customary, Prevailing and Reasonable; Fee Schedule Amount.*

American Medical Association (AMA): A voluntary membership association of physicians that is viewed as the main body responsible for speaking for physicians' concerns.

Annual Deductible: *See Deductible.*

Approved Charge: *See Allowable Charge.*

Assignment: A provider's agreement to accept Medicare's allowable charge as payment in full; accepting assignment constitutes a guarantee not to balance bill. *See also Balance Bill; Nonparticipating Physician; Participating Physician.*

Assistant-At-Surgery: An individual who has the necessary qualifications to participate in a particular operation and actively assists in performing the surgery.

Audit: An activity carried out by carriers and other Medicare agencies to determine the appropriateness and accuracy of a physician's charges and billing patterns.

Balance Bill: Billing the beneficiary for any fee in excess of that allowed by the insurance carrier. For Medicare, the amount the physician can balance bill is capped by the limiting charge. *See also Limiting Charge.*

Beneficiary: A person eligible to receive benefits under an insurance plan.

Capitation: A census-driven reimbursement system wherein a health plan provides medical services for a fixed monthly fee. Contracting providers may be reimbursed in the same manner.

Carrier: A private insurance company that contracts with the Health Care Financing Administration to administer claims for Medicare Part B services. Also commonly used to refer to any insurance company. *See also Medicare Part B.*

CF: *See Conversion Factor.*

CHAMPUS (Civilian Health and Medical Program of the Uniformed Services): A federally funded comprehensive health benefits program designed to provide coverage for armed forces personnel who receive care outside a military treatment facility.

Claim: A demand to the carrier, by the insured person, for payment of benefits under a policy.

Claim Form: A form used to present claim information in an organized manner to the carrier or intermediary. *See also HCFA-1500; UB-92.*

COB: *See Coordination of Benefits.*

Coding: A mechanism for identifying and defining services, procedures, and diagnoses.

Coinsurance: The portion of covered medical expenses that a beneficiary must pay after payment of the deductible. Under Medicare Part B, the beneficiary pays coinsurance of 20 percent of the allowable charges. Also called copayment. *See also Deductible.*

Competitive Medical Plan (CMP): A health plan that is eligible by law to enter into a Medicare contract in return for a capitation payment, but does not satisfy the requirements to be a federally qualified HMO. *See also Capitation; Federally Qualified HMO.*

Comprehensive Medical Insurance: A policy designed to give the protection offered by both a basic and a major medical health insurance policy.

Conversion Factor (CF): The number by which the relative value of a service is multiplied to establish a schedule of fees for physician payment. The conversion factor is a dollar amount. *See also Relative Value Scale; Medicare Fee Schedule.*

Coordination of Benefits (COB): An insurance plan provision that ensures that benefits paid to a patient covered under more than one group plan will be limited to 100 percent of the actual charge.

Copayment: *See Coinsurance.*

Cost Sharing: Where the beneficiary pays a portion of health expenses through deductibles and coinsurance; the rationale being that, since the beneficiary must share in the cost of the service, he will be a better consumer of health care services. *See also Coinsurance; Deductible.*

Covered Services: Services and procedures for which Medicare will pay.

CPR: *See Customary, Prevailing and Reasonable.*

CPT: *See Current Procedural Terminology.*

Cross-Over Patient: A patient who has both Medicare and Medicaid coverage. *See also Dual Eligibles.*

Current Procedural Terminology (CPT): A system of numerical codes and narrative descriptions published annually by the American Medical Association; it is used to code procedures and services, including office visits, X-rays, lab work, diagnostic services and procedures, and surgical procedures. This coding system is accepted by virtually all commercial insurance carriers and is required by Medicare and Medicaid. *See also Coding, HCFA'S Common Procedure Coding System (HCPCS).*

Customary Charge: Calculation of the physician's median charge for a service over a 12-month period. *See also Customary, Prevailing and Reasonable.*

Customary, Prevailing, and Reasonable (CPR): A Medicare designation for physician payment for services provided prior to January 1, 1992. Under CPR, payment for a service is limited to the lowest of (1) the physician's billed (or actual) charge for the service, (2) the physician's customary charge for the service, or (3) the prevailing charge for that service in the community. This designation is similar to the usual, customary, and reasonable (UCR) used by private insurers. *See also Usual, Customary, and Reasonable.*

Deductible: An established amount that the insured person must pay toward the cost of medical treatment before the benefits of the program go into effect. Medicare Part A has a hospital deductible of $736 per benefit period for 1996. Medicare Part B has an annual deductible of $100 for 1996.

Department of Health and Human Services (DHHS): The department of the U.S. government that is responsible for setting and administering policy on health programs.

Dependents: The spouse and children of the insured as defined in the insurance contract.

Diagnosis Related Groups (DRG): A system of classifying medical cases for payment based on primary diagnosis, secondary diagnosis, surgical procedures, age, sex, and presence of complications; used by Medicare for calculating payment of inpatient hospital services.

Direct Contract HMO: A HMO that contracts directly with individual physicians to provide services to enrolled members. *See also Health Maintenance Organization.*

Disability Income Insurance: A form of health insurance that provides periodic payments to replace income when the insured is unable to work as a result of illness, injury, or disease.

Disabled: As defined by the Social Security Administration, disabled refers to a person with a mental or physical impairment that keeps him from working and that is expected to last one year or more or to result in death.

Downcoding: A process used by carriers to reduce the allowable amount of billed procedures by changing the codes submitted to ones of lower value.

Dual Eligibles: Medicare beneficiaries who also receive the full range of Medicaid benefits offered in their state. *See also Cross-Over Patient.*

Durable Medical Equipment Regional Carrier (DMERC): A private insurance company that contracts with the Health Care Financing Administration to process Medicare claims for durable medical equipment, prosthetics, orthotics, and supplies. There are four regional carriers.

Electronic Claim: A claim form that is processed and delivered from one computer to another via some form of magnetic media (magnetic tape, diskette) or via telecommunications (telephone link).

Enrollee: *See Insured.*

EOB: *See Explanation of Benefits.*

EOMB: *See Explanation of Medicare Benefits.*

Evaluation and Management Services: Cognitive or non-procedural services provided by most physicians for the purpose of diagnosing and treating diseases and counseling and evaluating patients.

Exclusions: Specific services or conditions that a policy will not cover or covers at a limited rate.

Explanation of Benefits (EOB): A form from the insurance carrier that explains the benefits that were paid and/or charges that were rejected.

Explanation of Medicare Benefits (EOMB). The EOB form from the Medicare carrier. *See also Explanation of Benefits.*

Federally Qualified HMO: A HMO that has satisfied certain federal qualifications pertaining to organizational structure, provider contracts, health service delivery information, utilization review/quality assurance, grievance procedures, financial status, and marketing information.

Fee-For-Service: Payment system by which health care providers are paid for individual services rendered. UCR, CPR, and Fee Schedules are examples of fee-for-service systems. *See also Customary, Prevailing and Reasonable; Fee Schedule; Usual, Customary and Reasonable.*

Fee Schedule: A list of predetermined charges for medical services. *See also Medicare Fee Schedule.*

Fee Schedule Amount: The payment amount for a particular procedure, service, or supply as determined by the fee schedule. *Also called* Allowable. (Note: In this book, the term "allowable" is used to mean the fee schedule amount or otherwise established payment amount *as determined by Medicare.*)

Fee Schedule Payment Areas: Geographic areas within which payment under the fee schedule will be equal. *See also Geographic Adjustment Factor.*

Fiscal Intermediary (FI): A private insurance company that contracts with the Health Care Financing Administration to administer claims for Medicare Part A (e.g., hospital inpatient, skilled nursing facility) services and some Medicare Part B services (i.e., hospital outpatient department services). *See also Medicare Part A.*

Gaming: Gaining advantage by using improper means to evade the letter or intent of a rule or system.

Geographic Adjustment Factor (GAF): The adjustment made to a service's fee in the Medicare Fee Schedule to determine the correct payment in each fee schedule payment area.

Global Service: A group of clinically related services that are treated as a single unit for the purpose of coding, billing, and payment.

Group Practice HMO: A HMO that contracts with a multi-specialty physician group practice to provide all physician services to the HMO's enrollees. *See also Health Maintenance Organization.*

HCFA: *See Health Care Financing Administration.*

HCFA'S Common Procedure Coding System (HCPCS): A coding system developed by the Health Care Financing Administration as a supplement to CPT. Contains codes for nonphysician services, such as supplies, ambulance services, durable medical equipment and injections. *See also* Coding; Current Procedural Terminology.

HCFA-1500: A universal insurance claim form that is mandated for Medicare Part B billing and generally accepted by all insurance carriers.

Health Care Financing Administration (HCFA): The U.S. federal agency under the auspices of the Department of Health and Human Services with responsibility for administering the Medicare and Medicaid programs.

Health Insurance Claim Number (HICN): The 10-digit alpha-numeric assigned by the Health Care Financing Administration to each individual Medicare beneficiary; required on all claims and correspondence sent to Medicare. *Also called Medicare Number.*

Health Maintenance Organization (HMO): An organization that provides comprehensive health services to its members in return for a fixed prepaid fee. There are five types of HMOs: direct contract, group practice, independent physician association, network and staff. *See also* Direct Contract HMO; Group Practice HMO; Independent Physician Association HMO; Network HMO; Staff HMO.

Health Professional Shortage Area (HPSA): Areas designated by the Secretary of the Department of Health and Human Services as having a shortage of health care providers, including: (1) an urban or rural area (that need not conform to the geographic boundaries of a political subdivision and that is a rational area for the delivery of health services); (2) a population group; (3) a public nonprofit private medical facility. Designated HPSAs can apply for National Health Services Corps (NHSC) personnel or be eligible for the NHSC scholarship program or health profession student loan program.

HICN: *See Health Insurance Claim Number.*

HMO: *See Health Maintenance Organization.*

Indemnity Schedule: *See Schedule of Allowances.*

Independent Physician Association (IPA): A legal entity of individual independent physicians or small groups of physicians formed for the purpose of contracting with managed care organizations.

Independent Physician Association HMO: A HMO that contracts with an IPA to provide services to its members. Physicians can be members of the IPA for purposes of the HMO contract, but retain their practice separately. *See also Health Maintenance Organization; Independent Physician Association.*

Insured: The person who represents the family unit in relation to the insurance program. Usually the person whose employment makes coverage possible. *Also called* Enrollee, Policy Holder, and Subscriber.

Insurer: *See Carrier.*

International Classification of Diseases, Ninth Revision, Clinical Modification (ICD-9-CM): A system of numeric codes and narrative descriptions developed and maintained by the World Health Organization; used to code patient illnesses, injuries, symptoms, etc. This coding system is accepted by virtually all commercial insurance carriers and is required by Medicare and Medicaid. *See also Coding.*

Limited License Practitioner (LLP): A professional licensed to perform certain specific health care services in independent practice (e.g., podiatrists, dentists, optometrists, and chiropractors).

Limiting Charge: The maximum amount a nonparticipating physician is permitted to charge for a given service or procedure for which assignment is not accepted; calculated as 115 percent of the nonparticipating fee schedule amount. *See also Balance Bill.*

Long-Term Disability Income Insurance: A provision to pay benefits to a covered disabled person as long as he remains disabled, up to a specified period.

Medicaid: A program of health insurance for the poor and medically indigent. States share in financing the program with the federal government and determine eligibility and benefits consistent with federal standards.

Medicare: A federal health insurance program for people aged 65 or over, disabled persons, and persons with kidney failure.

Medicare Economic Index (MEI): An index that tracks changes over time in physician practice costs and general earnings levels.

Medicare Fee Schedule (MFS): The fee schedule used by Medicare to pay for physician services. This fee schedule, effective for services provided on or after January 1, 1992, is based on the resource costs of performing a procedure or service, including physician work, practice expense, and malpractice expense. Payment using the MFS is determined by multiplying the relative value units of a given procedure or service by the conversion factor. *See also Relative Value Scale; Conversion Factor.*

Medicare Part A: The Hospital Insurance program that covers the costs of hospital and related post-hospital services. It is available without payment of a premium to those who qualify under Social Security rules. Those not automatically eligible can purchase the coverage. Beneficiaries are responsible for an initial hospital deductible per incidence of illness and coinsurance for some services.

Medicare Part B: Medicare's Supplementary Medical Insurance program that covers the costs of physician services, outpatient surgery, outpatient lab and X-ray tests, durable medical equipment, and certain other services. As a voluntary program, Part B requires payment of a monthly premium. Beneficiaries are responsible for an annual deductible and coinsurance for most covered services.

Medigap Insurance: Health insurance policies offered by private carriers to cover the "gaps" in Medicare benefits, such as deductibles and coinsurance.

Modifiers: Codes that supplement CPT or HCPCS codes to indicate that the service has been changed in some way. *See also Current Procedural Terminology; HCFA'S Common Procedure Coding System.*

National Practitioner Data Bank: A permanent record, maintained by the U.S. Public Health Service, of disciplinary actions taken against physicians and all payments made on behalf of physicians for actual or potential malpractice claims.

Network HMO: A HMO that contracts with more than one group practice to provide physician services to the HMO's enrollees. Similar to the Group Practice HMO, except that more than one group practice is involved. *See also Health Maintenance Organization.*

No-Fault Insurance: Insurance that provides coverage against injury or loss without the need to determine responsibility for an accident.

Nonpar: *See Nonparticipating Physician.*

Nonparticipating Physician: A physician who does not sign a Medicare participation agreement, and therefore is not obligated to accept assignment on all claims. *Also called* Nonpar. *See also Participating Physician.*

Office of the Inspector General (OIG): Department of the Health Care Financing Administration that has responsibility for detecting and prosecuting fraud and abuse in the Medicare and Medicaid programs.

Par: *See Participating Physician.*

Participating Physician: A physician who signs a participation agreement, agreeing to accept assignment on all Medicare claims for a period of one year. *Also called* Par.

Participating Physician and Supplier Program: A program that provides financial and administrative incentives for physicians and suppliers to agree in advance to accept assignment on all Medicare claims for a one-year period.

Peer Review Organization (PRO): An organization that reviews the medical necessity and the quality of care provided to Medicare beneficiaries.

Physician Payment Review Commission (PPRC): A special commission that reports to Congress on the economics of health care services funded by the federal government.

PIN: *See Provider Identification Number.*

Policy Holder: *See Insured.*

PPO: *See Preferred Provider Organization.*

Preauthorization: *See Precertification.*

Precertification: The process of obtaining permission for a service from the insurance carrier before the service is performed. *Also called* Preauthorization.

Predetermination: The process of obtaining an estimate of what an insurance carrier will pay for service(s) before the service(s) is(are) performed.

Preferred Provider Organization (PPO): An entity through which an employer group health plan and insurers contract to purchase health care services from a selected group of participating providers. Contractual relationships are established by the employer with the "preferred" providers who agree to certain discounts in return for incentives, such as volume guarantees and prompt payment. Subscribers are offered financial incentives such as reduced deductible if they use the preferred providers. Penalties for using other providers can exist, such as higher coinsurance.

Premium: An amount paid periodically to purchase medical insurance benefits; for Medicare Part B services in 1996, beneficiaries must pay a premium of $42.50 per month.

Prevailing Charge: Charge calculated as a percent of customary charges of all physicians in a given locality. *See also Customary Charge; Customary, Prevailing and Reasonable.*

Primary Payer: The insurance carrier that has first responsibility for payment of benefits under Coordination of Benefits. *See also Coordination of Benefits; Secondary Payer.*

PRO: *See Peer Review Organization.*

Professional Component: The part of the relative value or fee for a procedure that represents physician work.

Professional Liability Insurance: The insurance physicians purchase to help protect themselves from the financial risks associated with malpractice claims and awards.

Provider: The person or other entity, such as a physician, limited license practitioner, supplier, or hospital, who provides services and supplies to the beneficiary.

Provider Identification Number (PIN): The number assigned by individual carriers to identify physicians and group practices that submit claims for Medicare services.

Qualified Medicare Beneficiary (QMB): A person who is entitled to Medicare Part A, has monthly income below

$665 in 1996 (or $884 for a family of two in 1996), and whose resources (not including personal home, automobile, burial plot, furniture, jewelry, and life insurance) do not exceed $4,000 in 1996 (or $6,000 for a couple in 1996). If a person meets these requirements, he can be entitled to have Medicaid pay his Medicare premiums, deductibles and coinsurance.

Railroad Retirement Board (RRB): The U.S. federal agency with responsibility for administering the Railroad Retirement program for railroad workers.

RBRVS: *See Resource Based Relative Value Scale.*

Reasonable Charge: For services provided prior to January 1, 1992, the reasonable charge was the amount Medicare would pay for a covered service. It was the lowest of the actual, customary, and prevailing charges.

Relative Value Scale: An index that assigns specific numeric values to medical services. Multiplying the relative value by a conversion factor results in a fee. *See also Conversion Factor.*

Relative Value Unit (RVU): A unit of measurement assigned to each procedure/service in a relative value scale.

Release of Information: The patient's signature indicating consent to the release of information necessary for settlement of an insurance claim.

Resource Based Relative Value Scale (RBRVS): A government-mandated relative value scale that is the basis for the Medicare Fee Schedule.

RRB: *See Railroad Retirement Board.*

RVU: *See Relative Value Unit.*

Schedule of Allowances: A list of specific amounts a carrier will pay toward the cost of medical services provided. *Also called Indemnity Schedule.*

Secondary Payer: The insurance carrier second in responsibility for payment of benefits under Coordination of Benefits. *See also Coordination of Benefits; Primary Payer.*

Social Security Administration (SSA): The U.S. federal agency with responsibility for administering the Social Security program.

Social Security Disability Benefits: Benefits paid to people with disabilities and their families.

Social Security Retirement Benefits: Benefits paid to people 62 or older and their families when worker retires.

Social Security Survivors Benefits: Benefits paid to families of workers who have died.

Specified Low Income Medicare Beneficiary (SLMB): A person who is entitled to Medicare Part A, has monthly income below $794 in 1996 (or $1,056 for a family of two in 1996), and whose resources (not including personal home, automobile, burial plot, furniture, jewelry, and life insurance) do not exceed $4,000 in 1996 (or $6,000 for a family of two in 1996). If a person meets these requirements, he can be entitled to have Medicaid pay for his Medicare Part B premiums.

SSA: *See Social Security Administration.*

SSI: *See Supplemental Security Income.*

Staff HMO: A HMO where the physicians are employed by the HMO. The physicians are usually paid a salary and may receive bonuses or incentives based on productivity and performance. *See also Health Maintenance Organization.*

Subscriber: *See Insured.*

Superbill: A multi-part pre-printed form that provides sufficient information so that patients may file their own insurance claim forms.

Supplemental Security Income (SSI): Income provided by the federal government for people aged 65 or older, blind or disabled who are low-income and who do not have substantial assets. People who qualify for SSI also usually qualify for food stamps and Medicaid benefits.

Supplier: Providers, other than practitioners, of health care services. Suppliers under Medicare include independent labs, durable medical equipment providers, ambulance services, orthotists, prosthetists, and portable X-ray providers.

Technical Component: The part of the relative value or fee for a procedure that represents the costs of performing the procedure, excluding physician work.

UB-92: A claim form that is mandated for billing Medicare Part A services.

UCR: *See Usual, Customary and Reasonable.*

Unbundling: The process of coding, billing, and requesting payment for single services that are generally included in a global charge. *See also Global Service.*

Unique Physician Identification Number (UPIN): A code number assigned by the Health Care Financing Administration to individual physicians; used to identify individual physicians who order or refer tests for Medicare beneficiaries.

Usual, Customary, and Reasonable (UCR): A method used by commercial insurers to establish payment for services. Comparable to Medicare's customary, prevailing, and reasonable. Insurers typically pay the lesser of the actual charge or the established UCR amount. *See also Customary, Prevailing and Reasonable.*

Utilization Review: The process of reviewing services provided to determine if those services were medically necessary and appropriate.

Volume Performance Standard (VPS): A federally established mechanism to adjust physician fees under the Medicare Fee Schedule based on how annual increases in actual expenditures compare to previously determined performance standard rates of increase.

Workers' Compensation: Payment of medical expenses and income support for employees who are injured during performance of or as a result of their work or who become ill as a result of their work. Coverage varies by state.

CHAPTER 1

MEDICARE ENTITLEMENT

To collect payment from Medicare, a person must be eligible for and enrolled in the Medicare program. Most of us take it for granted that all people over age 65 receive Medicare benefits—this is not necessarily true. An individual can elect not to receive the benefits or may not be eligible under the rules of the program. This chapter provides information about who is entitled to Medicare benefits and how and when to sign up to receive these benefits.

GENERAL ENTITLEMENT

When individuals reach the age of 65 and are eligible for Social Security retirement or survivor benefits or Railroad Retirement benefits, they are eligible for Medicare benefits. For those eligible for retirement benefits, Part A benefits are provided free of charge (called premium-free). Hospital insurance benefits are also available to persons under age 65 if they have received Social Security or Railroad Retirement disability benefits for 24 months, or if they have end stage renal disease (ESRD). Part B benefits are available to all persons aged 65 or over, regardless of eligibility for Social Security benefits.

Most people aged 65 or over who are not eligible for Social Security retirement benefits can voluntarily enroll for hospital insurance (Part A) coverage if they are:

- 65 or over;

- live in the United States; *and*

- are a citizen of the U.S., or an alien legally admitted to the U.S.

Voluntary enrollees are required to pay a monthly premium for this coverage; for 1996, those premiums are $289 or $188 per month, depending upon the number of quarter-of-coverage credits earned. All beneficiaries are required to pay a deductible amount of $736 for each hospital benefit period (see "Benefit Period" below) and coinsurance for hospital stays in excess of 60 days.

Unlike premium-free Part A, Part B requires that all enrollees pay a monthly premium for their benefits. For calendar year 1996, the Part B premium is $42.50 per month. Part B enrollees also pay coinsurance and a yearly deductible. The 1996 deductible is $100 and the coinsurance amount is 20 percent of Medicare's allowable charge.

Part B benefits are available to all resident citizens (and certain aliens) aged 65 or over, even to those not eligible for Social Security or Railroad Retirement benefits. Medical insurance benefits are also available to persons under age 65 if they have been receiving Social Security or Railroad Retirement disability benefits for 24 months, or if they have ESRD.

Three different categories of people are entitled to Medicare benefits. Some facts about these groups, and their specific requirements for entitlement, are discussed on the following pages.

Over Age 65

- A person eligible for benefits based on age is considered eligible on the first day of the month he reaches age 65 and is eligible for Social Security or Railroad Retirement benefits.

- An entitled person's spouse or surviving spouse who is over age 65 is also eligible for benefits on the basis of the spouse's entitlement.

- Entitlement continues until death or until the enrollee notifies Medicare in writing of his wish to terminate coverage.

Disabled

- People who are entitled to Social Security benefits or Railroad Retirement benefits due to disability are also entitled to Medicare benefits. To obtain Medicare coverage, the person seeking benefits must be fully insured and insured for disability coverage (see "Determining Your Entitlement").

- Entitlement under Social Security disability also extends to disabled widows and widowers between the ages of 50 and 65, and persons aged 18 and over who receive Social Security benefits because they became disabled prior to reaching age 22.

- Persons over the age of 65 cannot receive Medicare benefits under the disability provision because benefits are available under the over age 65 provision.

- Of the 37.5 million beneficiaries entitled to
  Medicare, only 11.7 percent, or 4.4 million people
  are entitled on the basis of disability.

Coverage under this category begins 24 months after
the insured becomes entitled to Social Security benefits.
Entitlement begins the first day of the 25th month of
disability entitlement and terminates at the end of the month
following the month disability entitlement ends (or at the
end of the month prior to the month the individual reaches
age 65).

However, there is a five-month waiting period to obtain
coverage, which means the beneficiary cannot receive
benefits for 29 months after becoming disabled. Entitlement
ends the last day of the month following the month the
beneficiary is notified of the disability termination, or the
last day of the month before the month in which the
beneficiary reaches age 65.

Certain special circumstances can extend Medicare
entitlement for Medicare beneficiaries who attempt to return
to work or who give up their disability status for other
reasons. These include:

- For a beneficiary who returns to work, coverage
  can be continued during a nine-month period of
  "trial work" and for up to 15 months thereafter, for
  a total of 24 months.

- For a beneficiary who returns to work or loses his
  disability status for other reasons, he can regain
  Medicare entitlement without being subject to the
  24-month waiting period as long as the second
  disability is the same as or directly related to the
  first disability. If the second disability is unrelated

to the first, the 24-month waiting period can still be avoided if the worker returns to disability status within 60 months after the first disability or the beneficiary (other than the worker, such as a widow or widower) returns to disability status within 84 months.

End Stage Renal Disease

Individuals who have ESRD are entitled to Medicare coverage if they are:

- entitled to monthly Social Security or Railroad Retirement benefits; or

- currently insured for old-age and survivors benefits; *or*

- spouses or dependents of entitled individuals.

For example, if a person is under age 65 and has reached currently or fully insured status (see "Determining Your Entitlement") or is receiving monthly Social Security benefits and has ESRD, he is entitled to Medicare coverage. His dependent(s) are covered only if they also have ESRD. Medicare also covers the costs of care for actual or potential kidney donors, including all reasonable preoperative, operative, and postoperative recovery expenses (postoperative payments are only for the actual period of recovery).

Regular Part A and Part B coverage are available to these participants; coverage is not limited to the treatment of the renal disease.

During the first 18 months of entitlement, beneficiaries who also have coverage through an employer group health plan will receive only secondary benefits from Medicare. Medicare entitlement begins the first day of the third month after the month in which the individual begins a course of renal dialysis. Individuals who participate in a self-dialysis training course may become eligible prior to the regular three-month waiting period.

For those who are candidates for a kidney transplant, coverage may begin as early as the first day of the month in which the individual is hospitalized for the transplant, providing the surgery takes place within two months of hospitalization. Individuals who received a transplant that failed and who have initiated another course of dialysis are again entitled to benefits as of the first day of the month in which the course of dialysis begins.

For transplant recipients, coverage ends three years (the last day of the 36th month) after the month of the transplant. For individuals who do not receive a kidney transplant, coverage ends the last day of the 12th month after the month in which a regular course of dialysis was ended. Medicare maintains only about 226,000 beneficiaries under this classification.

Government Employees

Medicare Part A coverage for government employees was not available until 1983 (unless they were eligible on the basis of employment in the private sector or as a spouse of a retired or disabled worker). Offered in two stages, Medicare coverage was first extended to federal employees, who were required to begin paying FICA tax. State and local government employees hired after March 31, 1986, later became eligible for coverage and began paying the FICA tax.

The Tax Equity and Fiscal Responsibility Act of 1982 provided a transitional provision for federal government employees who would retire and therefore not earn enough quarters of coverage before retirement to be entitled to Medicare. The provision allowed federal employees to have their federal employment during and before January 1983 treated like private employment for purposes of credit toward Medicare eligibility (up to the minimum number of quarters required).

Some government employment is not Medicare-qualified, which means that the employment is not counted toward Medicare eligibility. Those federal government employees whose employment is *not* Medicare-qualified include:

- Inmates in federal penal institutions.

- Interns (other than medical or dental interns or medical or dental residents in training) and student nurses employed by the federal government.

- Employees serving on a temporary basis in case of fire, storm, earthquake, flood, or similar emergency.

Those state and local government employees whose employment is *not* Medicare-qualified include:

- Individuals employed to relieve them from unemployment.

- Patients or inmates in a hospital, home, or other institution.

- Employees serving on a temporary basis in case of fire, storm, snow, earthquake, flood, or similar emergency.

- Interns (other than medical or dental interns or medical or dental residents in training), student nurses, and other student employees of hospitals in the District of Columbia.

- Election officials or election workers, if the remuneration for services performed in a calendar year is less than $1,000.

DETERMINING YOUR ENTITLEMENT

Usually, an individual who applies for and establishes entitlement for Social Security retirement or Railroad Retirement benefits is considered to have also filed for Medicare benefits. A person who is entitled to Social Security benefits but who does not file an application for benefits must do so to enroll for hospital insurance benefits.

Upon establishing eligibility and enrolling for Part A, the individual is automatically enrolled in Part B. An individual can enroll in Part A but refuse Part B benefits, which he indicates when filing his application for benefits. However, individuals who purchase Part A must also enroll in Part B.

Railroad Retirement Entitlement

Being entitled to Railroad Retirement benefits generally means the person is entitled to an annuity or a pension under the Railroad Retirement Act. This entitlement to Railroad Retirement benefits also entitles the enrollee to Medicare benefits.

The Railroad Retirement Board (RRB) and the Health Care Financing Administration (HCFA) have an agreement regarding responsibilities of Railroad Retirement beneficiaries and the Medicare Part B program. Under this agreement, the RRB is responsible for:

- Enrolling those eligible for Railroad Retirement benefits in Part B.

- Collecting Part B premiums from Railroad Retirement beneficiaries.

- Selecting carriers to process Railroad Retirement beneficiaries' Part B claims.

The RRB selected the Travelers Insurance Company to act as the carrier for railroad beneficiaries, regardless of where the services are furnished. RRB is required, through its carrier, to apply the same policies and regulations as HCFA in making coverage and payment determinations.

Social Security Entitlement

To determine whether you are eligible for Social Security retirement benefits and therefore for Medicare benefits, you need to determine whether you or your spouse have earned enough quarter of coverage credits. *It is important to note that, while you can be eligible for and receive Social Security retirement benefits at age 62, you will have to reach age 65 before you can receive Medicare benefits.*

Quarters of Coverage

To find out whether you are eligible for Social Security retirement benefits, you must determine whether you are "fully insured," meaning you have accumulated a sufficient number of "quarters of coverage credits." A quarter is defined as a three-month period beginning January 1, April 1, July 1, or October 1.

Most employed workers before 1978 were awarded one quarter of coverage for each calendar quarter in which they were paid $50 or more in wages. (For Social Security and Medicare purposes, *worker* refers to either you or the person upon whose earnings record you depend to establish entitlement to Social Security retirement benefits.) A self-employed person with $400 or more of net earnings in a year got four quarters of coverage for that year. Farm workers got one quarter of coverage for each $100 of cash wages paid to them in a year, up to a maximum of four.

Congress changed the method of calculating quarters of coverage beginning in 1978. Now, workers get one quarter of coverage for a set amount of earnings in a year, up to a maximum of four quarters. For 1978, the set amount was $250. Thus, earnings of $1,000 in 1978 gained four quarters of coverage, even if all the wages were paid in one quarter.

For 1996, the quarter of coverage amount is $640. Thus, earnings of $2,560 gain four quarters of coverage, even if all the wages are paid in one quarter. However, in the case of the self-employed person, annual net earnings of at least $400 continued to be required before any quarters could be credited.

Qualification for disability benefits is different. If you become severely disabled, you are eligible for monthly benefits if you have worked under Social Security long enough and recently enough. The amount of work you will need depends on your age when you became disabled:

- *Before age 24:* You need credit for 1½ years of work (6 quarters of coverage) in the three-year period ending when your disability began.

- *Age 24 through 30:* You need credit for having worked half of the time since you were age 21 until the time you became disabled.

- *Age 31 or older:* All workers disabled at age 31 or older—except the blind—need the amount of credit shown in Figure 1-1 below.

Figure 1-1: Work Credit for Disability Benefits[*]

Born after 1929; became disabled at age:	Born before 1930; became disabled before age 62 in:	Years you need:
42 or younger	1971	5
44	1973	5½
46	1975	6
48	1977	6½
50	1979	7
52	1981	7½
54	1983	8
56	1985	8½
58	1987	9
60	1989	9½
62 or older	1991 or later	10

[*] *©Commerce Clearing House, 1996 Medicare Explained*

Five years of this credit must have been earned in the ten years ending when the worker became disabled. The years need not be continuous or in units of full years.

Fully Insured

To qualify for Social Security retirement benefits, a worker must be *fully insured*; this status is required for other major types of benefits as well. Forty quarters of coverage will fully insure any worker for life, so that a worker with 10 years of work in jobs covered by Social Security can assume that he is covered.

Due to changes in the Social Security law and the inclusion of certain workers who had previously been excluded from Social Security coverage, some people may be able to earn fewer than 40 quarters to be considered fully insured. Persons near retirement age can use the table in Figure 1-2 to determine the necessary number of quarters of coverage to be considered fully insured.

Currently Insured

A minimum of six quarters of coverage is required to be paid any benefits. Certain kinds of benefits are payable when the worker is only *currently insured*, meaning that he has at least six quarters of coverage (but not enough to be fully insured) in the 13-quarter period ending with the quarter in which he becomes entitled to retirement benefits, disability benefits, or dies. The table in Figure 1-3 shows how the worker must be insured to qualify for entitlement to each type of benefit.

Figure 1-2: Quarters of Coverage Needed

Year Worker Reaches Age 62	Quarters Needed to Be Fully Insured
1987	36
1988	37
1989	38
1990	39
1991 or later	40

Special rules apply for *employees of nonprofit organizations* brought into the system beginning in 1984:

Age as of January 1, 1984	Quarters Needed to Be Fully Insured
60 or older	6
59	8
58	12
57	16
55 or 56	20

ENROLLING IN SOCIAL SECURITY AND MEDICARE

If you are age 62 or older and have retired, you need to enroll for Social Security retirement benefits, which will also enroll you for Medicare benefits (which you will receive when you turn 65). To do this, make an appointment with your local Social Security office.

You will meet with an adviser who will ask you a series of questions. Your answers will be input into the Social Security Administration's computer system. Some of the information you will be asked for by the Social Security Administration includes:

• Name, including maiden name (if applicable).

- Social Security number.

- Date of birth.

- State or country of birth.

- Current disabilities, including the date of disability.

- Whether you have ever filed an application for benefits, or someone has filed one on your behalf, including Social Security number of person on whose record you filed other application.

- Active military service history after September 7, 1939 and before 1968, including dates of service.

- Current or past eligibility for monthly benefit from a military or civilian federal agency (including VA benefits only if you waived military retirement pay).

- Whether you or your spouse worked in the railroad industry for seven years or more.

- Current and past marital status, including name and Social Security number of current spouse, date and place (city and state) of marriage, whether marriage was performed by clergy, public official, or other person, how marriage ended (if divorced).

- Whether you wish this application to protect your spouse's right to Social Security benefits.

Figure 1-3: Entitlement Requirements

Retirement Benefits	Requirement
Retired worker, age 62+	Fully insured
Spouse, or divorced spouse, age 62+	Fully insured
Spouse, any age, if caring for child entitled to benefits	Fully insured
Child or grandchild under 18, under 19 if student, or any age if disabled	Fully insured

Survivors Benefits	Requirement
Widow, widower, or divorced person, age 60 or over, or 50-59 and disabled	Fully insured
Widow, divorced parent of deceased worker's child, or widower, any age, caring for a young child entitled to benefits	Either fully or currently insured
Child or grandchild under age 18, under 19 if student, or any age if disabled	Either fully or currently insured
Dependent parent, age 62+	Fully insured

- Name(s) of children under age 18 who are dependent upon you.

- Company(ies) for which you have worked within the last two years.

- Permission to contact your employer(s) for wage information.

- Whether you are an officer of a corporation or related to an officer of a corporation.

- Whether you were self-employed this year, last year, or the year before, including the type of trade or business.

- Total earnings last year.

- Expected earnings this year.

- Expected earnings next year.

- Annual report of earnings if you expect to make any money this year or next.

- When you want your benefits to begin.

- Whether you wish to enroll in Part B Medicare.

- If born after January 2, 1924 whether you expect to be entitled to a pension or annuity based on work after 1956 not covered by Social Security, including date of entitlement or eligibility.

- Whether you want your benefit check direct deposited.

- Signature.

- Address, city, state, zip code.

- Telephone number.

It will take approximately 40-60 minutes to complete this process if you are prepared. Enrollment in Medicare Part A is automatic when you complete the questions. Enrollment in Part B is accomplished by saying "Yes" when asked if you want to enroll in the Supplemental Medical Insurance program. If you do not want Part B, indicate this choice by saying "No" when asked. Note, however, that if you elect not to have Part B coverage, your premium for this coverage will be higher should you sign up for Part B at a later date, unless you have coverage through your or your spouse's employer's group coverage. (See "Special Enrollment.")

Documents Needed

You will need to bring the following documents when you apply for benefits:

- The *Social Security number* of the person on whose work record you are applying, whether that is your own, or your spouse's, or other person's on whom you are dependent. You can present your Social Security card or report the number if you have lost your card.

- *Proof of age*, ideally a birth or baptismal certificate. Alternate proofs of age such as a passport, a census record, school records, marriage certificate, life insurance policy, family bible with birth dates, or any other document that establishes your age may be acceptable. If there is some question about your age, bring as many of these documents as possible. If your original birth certificate is wrong, bring the corrected certificate or other documents that establish your correct age as well as those documents that show your attempt(s) to correct your original birth certificate.

- Your *marriage certificate, divorce decree and/or death certificate*, if you are applying as a dependent or surviving spouse.

- Your *children's birth certificates and Social Security numbers*, if you are applying for them as dependents or survivors.

- The *W-2 forms*, or federal income tax returns if self-employed, for the previous two years for the person on whose earnings record you are claiming benefits.

- *Proof of military service*, if any, since extra work credits may be given for active military duty.

Enrollment

As discussed above, you enroll for Medicare benefits at the same time you enroll for Social Security benefits. You can file an application for Social Security benefits as early as three months before you reach age 62 or at any time after that. To guarantee your Medicare entitlement is effective when you turn 65, be sure to file for benefits at the beginning of your initial enrollment period, which begins three months before you reach age 65.

Enrollment in Parts A and B is automatic when you complete the form for Social Security benefits, unless you indicate your choice not to have Part B coverage at that time. If you receive Social Security benefits prior to turning 65, your enrollment in Medicare will be automatic when you turn 65; you do not need to file an application or notify Social Security or Medicare of your eligibility.

If you are disabled, you will automatically be enrolled in Medicare when you have been a Social Security disability beneficiary for 24 months.

If you want to wait to receive your Social Security benefits after you turn 65 (for example, because you are currently employed), but you want Medicare benefits to start at age 65, you will need to file an application to enroll for Medicare benefits.

You must apply for Medicare benefits if you: are planning to work past age 65; are age 65 but not eligible for premium-free Part A benefits; or have permanent kidney failure.

Please note that if you are not eligible for premium-free Part A and you decide to enroll in this program, you will also have to enroll in Part B, at a total cost of $331.50 per month (1996). You can enroll in Part B without enrolling in Part A but you cannot enroll in Part A without Part B (when you do not qualify for premium-free benefits).

To file for benefits, you must complete HCFA Form 18F5 "Application for Hospital Insurance Entitlement," a copy of which is shown in Figure 1-4. Please note this form

Figure 1-4: Form 18F5 — Application for Hospital Insurance Entitlement (page 1)

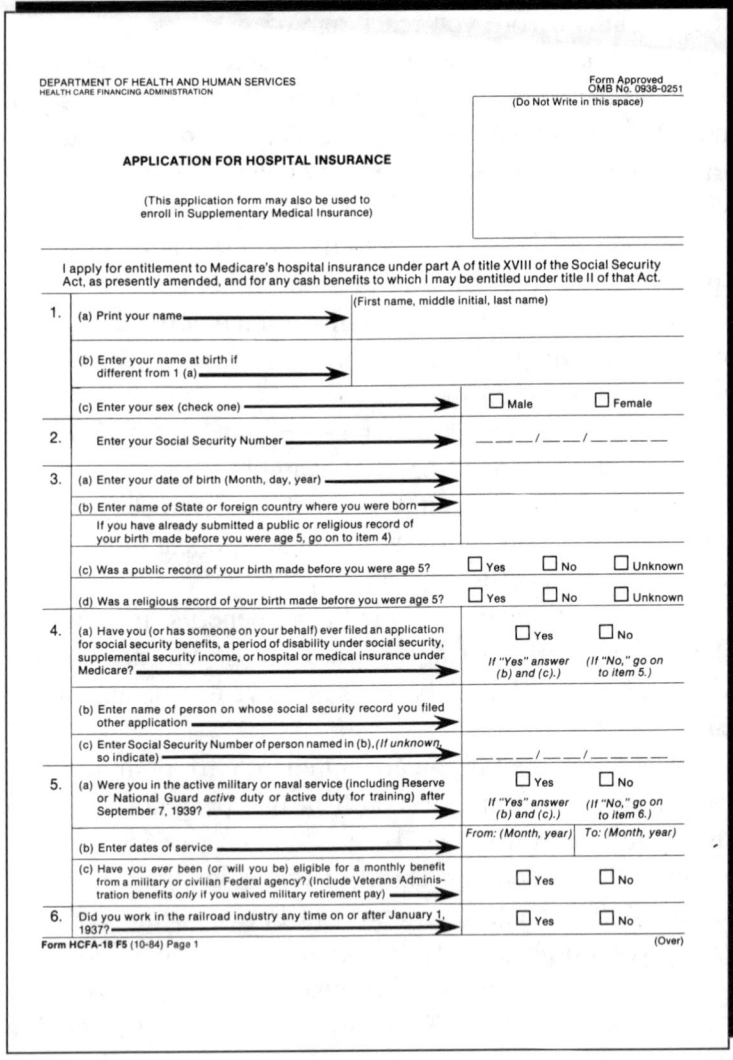

DEPARTMENT OF HEALTH AND HUMAN SERVICES
HEALTH CARE FINANCING ADMINISTRATION

Form Approved
OMB No. 0938-0251

(Do Not Write in this space)

APPLICATION FOR HOSPITAL INSURANCE

(This application form may also be used to
enroll in Supplementary Medical Insurance)

I apply for entitlement to Medicare's hospital insurance under part A of title XVIII of the Social Security
Act, as presently amended, and for any cash benefits to which I may be entitled under title II of that Act.

1. (a) Print your name ────────► (First name, middle initial, last name)

   (b) Enter your name at birth if
   different from 1 (a) ────────►

   (c) Enter your sex (check one) ────────► ☐ Male   ☐ Female

2. Enter your Social Security Number ────────► ___ ___ / ___ ___ / ___ ___ ___ ___

3. (a) Enter your date of birth (Month, day, year) ────────►

   (b) Enter name of State or foreign country where you were born ────►
   If you have already submitted a public or religious record of
   your birth made before you were age 5, go on to item 4)

   (c) Was a public record of your birth made before you were age 5?   ☐ Yes   ☐ No   ☐ Unknown

   (d) Was a religious record of your birth made before you were age 5?   ☐ Yes   ☐ No   ☐ Unknown

4. (a) Have you (or has someone on your behalf) ever filed an application
   for social security benefits, a period of disability under social security,
   supplemental security income, or hospital or medical insurance under
   Medicare? ────────►
   ☐ Yes   ☐ No
   If "Yes" answer   (If "No," go on
   (b) and (c).)   to item 5.)

   (b) Enter name of person on whose social security record you filed
   other application ────────►

   (c) Enter Social Security Number of person named in (b), (If unknown,
   so indicate) ────────►   ___ ___ / ___ ___ / ___ ___ ___ ___

5. (a) Were you in the active military or naval service (including Reserve
   or National Guard active duty or active duty for training) after
   September 7, 1939? ────────►
   ☐ Yes   ☐ No
   If "Yes" answer   (If "No," go on
   (b) and (c).)   to item 6.)

   (b) Enter dates of service ────────►
   From: (Month, year)   To: (Month, year)

   (c) Have you ever been (or will you be) eligible for a monthly benefit
   from a military or civilian Federal agency? (Include Veterans Administration benefits only if you waived military retirement pay) ────────►
   ☐ Yes   ☐ No

6. Did you work in the railroad industry any time on or after January 1,
   1937? ────────►   ☐ Yes   ☐ No

Form HCFA-18 F5 (10-84) Page 1   (Over)

Figure 1-4 *continued*: Form 18F5 — Application for Hospital Insurance Entitlement (page 2)

7.	(a) Have you ever engaged in work that was covered under the social security system of a country other than the United States?	☐ Yes ☐ No
	(b) If "Yes," list the country(ies).	

8.	(a) How much were your total earnings last year (If none, write "None")	Earnings $
	(b) How much do you expect your total earnings to be this year? (If none, write "None")	Earnings $

9.	Are you a resident of the United States? (To reside in a place means to make a home there.)	☐ Yes ☐ No

10.	(a) Are you a citizen of the United States? (If "Yes," go on to item 11.) (If "No" answer (b) and (c) below.)	☐ Yes ☐ No
	(b) Are you lawfully admitted for permanent residence in the United States?	☐ Yes ☐ No

(c) Enter below the information requested about your place of residence in the last 5 years:

ADDRESS AT WHICH YOU RESIDED IN THE LAST 5 YEARS (Begin with the most recent address. Show actual date residence began even if that is prior to the last 5 years)	DATE RESIDENCE BEGAN			DATE RESIDENCE ENDED		
	Month	Day	Year	Month	Day	Year

(If you need more space, use the "Remarks" space on the third page or another sheet of paper)

11. YOUR CURRENT MARRIAGE	Are you currently married?	☐ Yes ☐ No
	(If "Yes," give the following information about your current marriage.) (If "No" go on to item 12.)	
	To whom married (Enter your wife's maiden name or your husband's name)	When (Month, day, year)
	Spouse's date of birth (or age)	Spouse's Social Security Number (If none or unknown, so indicate) __ __ __ / __ __ / __ __ __ __

12. YOUR PREVIOUS MARRIAGE	If you had a previous marriage and your spouse died, OR if you had a previous marriage which lasted 10 or more years, give the following information. (If you had no previous marriage (s), enter "NONE.")	
	To whom married (Enter your wife's maiden name or your husband's name).	When (Month, day, year)
	Spouse's date of birth (or age)	Spouse's Social Security Number (If none or unknown, so indicate) __ __ __ / __ __ / __ __ __ __
	If spouse deceased, give date of death	

(Use "Remarks" space on page 3 for information about any other marriages.)

Form HCFA-18 F5 (10-84) Page 2

Figure 1-4 *continued*: Form 18F5 — Application for Hospital
Insurance Entitlement (page 3)

13.	Is or was your spouse a railroad worker, railroad retirement pensioner, or a railroad retirement annuitant? ⟶	☐ Yes ☐ No
14.	(a) Were you or your spouse a civilian employee of the Federal Government after June 1960? ⟶ (If "Yes," answer (b).) (If "No," omit (b), (c), and (d).)	☐ Yes ☐ No
	(b) Are you or your spouse now covered under a medical insurance plan provided by the Federal Employees Health Benefits Act of 1959? (If "Yes," omit (c) and (d).) (If "No," answer (c).)	☐ Yes ☐ No
	(c) Are you **and** your spouse barred from coverage under the above Act because your Federal employment, or your spouse's was not long enough? If "Yes," omit (d) and explain in "Remarks" below.) (If "No," answer (d).)	☐ Yes ☐ No
	(d) Were either you or your spouse an employee of the Federal Government after February 15, 1965? ⟶	☐ Yes ☐ No

Remarks:

_____

_____

_____

_____

_____

_____

_____

| 15. | If you are found to be otherwise ineligible for hospital insurance under Medicare, do you wish to enroll for hospital insurance on a monthly premium basis (in addition to the monthly premium for supplementary medical insurance)? ⟶ (If "Yes," you MUST also sign up for medical insurance.) | ☐ Yes ☐ No |

INFORMATION ON MEDICAL INSURANCE UNDER MEDICARE

Medical insurance under Medicare helps pay your doctor bills. It also helps pay for a number of other medical items and services not covered under the hospital insurance part of Medicare.

If you sign up for medical insurance, you must pay a premium for each month you have this protection. If you get monthly social security, railroad retirement, or civil service benefits, your premium will be deducted from your benefit check, if you get none of these benefits, you will be notified how to pay your premium.

The Federal Government contributes to the cost of your insurance. The amount of your premium and the Government's payment are based on the cost of services covered by medical insurance. The Government also makes additional payments when necessary to meet the full cost of the program. (Currently, the Government pays about two-thirds of the cost of this program.) You will get advance notice if there is any change in your premium amount.

If you have questions or would like a leaflet on medical insurance, call any Social Security office.

SEE OTHER SIDE TO SIGN UP FOR MEDICAL INSURANCE

Form HCFA-18 F5 (10-84) Page 3   (Over)

Figure 1-4 *continued*: Form 18F5 — Application for Hospital Insurance Entitlement (page 4)

If you become entitled to hospital insurance as a result of this application, you will be enrolled for medical insurance automatically unless you indicate below that you do not want this protection. If you decline to enroll now, you can get medical insurance protection later only if you sign up for it during specified enrollment periods. Your protection may then be delayed and you may have to pay a higher premium when you decide to sign up.

The date your medical insurance begins and the amount of the premium you must pay depend on the month you file this application with the Social Security Administration. Any social security office will be glad to explain the rules regarding enrollment to you.

16.	**DO YOU WISH TO ENROLL FOR SUPPLEMENTARY MEDICAL INSURANCE?** ➤ *(If "Yes," answer question 17.)* *(Enrollees for premium hospital insurance must simultaneously enroll for medical insurance.)*	☐ Yes ☐ No ☐ Currently Enrolled
17.	Are you or your spouse receiving an annuity under the Federal Civil Service Retirement Act or other law administered by the Office of Personnel Management? ➤	☐ Yes ☐ No Your No.
	(If "Yes," enter Civil Service annuity number here. Include the prefix "CSA" for annuitant, "CSF" for survivor.)	Spouse's No.
	If you entered your spouse's number, is he (she) enrolled for supplementary medical insurance under social security? ➤	☐ Yes ☐ No

I know that anyone who makes or causes to be made a false statement or representation of material fact in an application or for use in determining a right to payment under the Social Security Act commits a crime punishable under Federal law by fine, imprisonment or both. I affirm that all information I have given in this document is true.

SIGNATURE OF APPLICANT	Date *(Month, day, year)*
Signature *(First name, middle initial, last name) (Write in Ink)* **SIGN HERE** ▶	Telephone Number(s) at which you may be contacted during the day

Mailing address *(Number and street, Apt. No., P.O. Box, or Rural Route)*

City and State	ZIP Code	Enter Name of County (if any) in which you now live

Witnesses are required ONLY if this application has been signed by mark (X) above. If signed by mark (X), two witnesses to the signing who know the applicant must sign below, giving their full addresses.

1. Signature of Witness	2. Signature of Witness
Address *(Number and street, City, State, and ZIP Code)*	Address *(Number and street, City, State, and ZIP Code)*

Form HCFA-18 F5 (10-84) Page 4   ✩ U.S. Government Printing Office: 1986—607-648

Figure 1-4 *continued*: Form 18F5 — Application for Hospital Insurance Entitlement (page 5)

A REMINDER TO APPLICANTS FOR THE SOCIAL SECURITY HOSPITAL INSURANCE

NAME OF PERSON TO CONTACT ABOUT YOUR CLAIM	SSA OFFICE	DATE

TELEPHONE NO.

RECEIPT FOR YOUR CLAIM

Your application for the hospital insurance has been received and will be processed as quickly as possible.

You should hear from us within _____ days after you have given us all the information we requested. Some claims may take longer if additional information is needed.

In the meantime, if you change your mailing address, you should report the change.

Always give us your claim number when writing or telephoning about your claim.

If you have any questions about your claim, we will be glad to help you.

CLAIMANT	SOCIAL SECURITY CLAIM NUMBER

COLLECTION AND USE OF INFORMATION FROM YOUR APPLICATION — PRIVACY ACT NOTICE

PRIVACY ACT NOTICE: The Social Security Administration (SSA) is authorized to collect the information on this form under sections 226 and 1818 of the Social Security Act, as amended (42 U.S.C. 426 and 1395-17) and section 103 of Public Law 89-97. The information on this form is needed to enable social security and the Health Care Financing Administration (HCFA) to determine if you and your dependents may be entitled to hospital and/or medical insurance coverage and/or monthly benefits. While you do not have to furnish the information requested on this form to social security, no benefits or hospital or medical insurance can be provided until an application has been received by a social security office. Failure to provide all or part of the information requested could prevent an accurate and timely decision on your claim or your dependent's claim, and could result in the loss of some benefits of hospital or medical insurance. Although the information you furnish on this form is almost never used for any other purpose than stated above, there is a possibility that for the administration of social security or HCFA programs or for the administration of programs requiring coordination with SSA or HCFA, information may be disclosed to another person or to another governmental agency as follows: 1) to enable a third party or an agency to assist social security or HCFA in establishing rights to social security benefits and/or hospital or medical insurance coverage; 2) to comply with Federal laws requiring the release of information from social security and HCFA records (e.g., to the General Accounting Office and the Veterans Administration); and 3) to facilitate statistical research and audit activities necessary to assure the integrity and improvement of the social security and HCFA programs (e.g., to the Bureau of the Census and private concerns under contract to social security and HCFA).

Form HCFA-18 F5 (10-84) Page 5

(and any application for Medicare benefits) must be completed by the person requesting the benefits *prior* to his death. A relative or legal representative cannot file for retroactive Medicare entitlement after the beneficiary's death.

Because of the high cost of the Part A component of Medicare, you may want to consider shopping around for less expensive coverage. Although it is unlikely, some commercial carriers may offer comparable insurance coverage at a lower rate, or additional benefits beyond what Medicare offers for the same cost.

Initial Enrollment Period

Initial enrollment may take place during the seven-month period that begins three months before the month in which you turn age 65 and ends three months after the month you turn age 65. If you fail to sign up for Medicare in the first three months of your initial enrollment period, your Part B coverage will be delayed one to three months after enrollment. Also, if you fail to enroll for benefits during your initial enrollment period, you may have to pay a higher premium for coverage (unless you delay enrollment due to coverage from an employer group health plan).

General Enrollment Period

If you have premium-free Part A benefits but do not have Medicare Part B, you can sign up for Part B during a general enrollment period. This runs from January 1 through March 31 of each year. Coverage then begins as of July 1 of that year.

If you did not sign up for Part B coverage when you established your Social Security and Part A entitlement, your monthly premium may be increased by 10 percent for each 12-month period you could have had Part B but were not enrolled. (If you are covered under your employer's or your spouses's employer's group health plan, this increase does not apply. See "Special Enrollment" below.)

Some people have not earned enough quarters of coverage to be fully insured and therefore do not receive Part A benefits free of charge. These people are required to pay a premium for Part A coverage.

If either you or your spouse has fewer than 30 quarters of coverage, your Part A premium is $289 per month in 1996. If either you or your spouse has 30 or more quarters of coverage but fewer than 40, your Part A premium is $188 per month in 1996.

You can enroll in Medicare Part A during the general enrollment period (January 1 - March 31). If you enroll during a general enrollment period that begins more than one year after you became eligible to buy Part A, your monthly premium may be 10 percent higher than the basic premium amount.

For those who continue to work, you can usually delay enrollment until you quit working without a penalty. Coverage begins July 1 of the year you enroll.

Special Enrollment Period

A special enrollment period has been established for those persons who have health insurance through their spouse's employer or who continue to work after age 65 and have health insurance through their employer.

If you are covered by a group health plan when you are first able to get Medicare, you may be able to delay enrollment in Part B or premium Part A without a premium penalty and without waiting for a general enrollment period.

The group health plan must be based on your (or your spouse's) current employment; it cannot be a plan for retirees.

You can sign up for Part B or premium Part A at any time while you are covered under a group health plan if: (1) you are 65 or over and your group health coverage is based on your own or your spouse's current employment; or (2) you are disabled and your group health coverage is based on your own or a family member's current employment. (Disabled persons may be able to continue under their employer's group health coverage or may be covered under their spouse's employer's group health coverage, even while they are disabled.)

If you chose to delay enrolling in Part B or premium Part A because you didn't need Medicare coverage while you were covered under a group health plan, you may enroll during a special eight-month period, which is the eight months following termination of the employer's coverage.

If you are 65 or over, special enrollment applies when your or your spouse's current employment ends or your coverage under the group health plan ends, whichever comes first.

If you are disabled, you may enroll when the current employment ends, the plan is no longer classifiable as a large group health plan (one that covers 100 or more employees), or the plan coverage is terminated, whichever comes first.

PAYMENT OF YOUR PREMIUM

If you are receiving Social Security retirement or Railroad Retirement benefits, your Part B premium will be deducted from your monthly check. For those who must pay a premium for Part A benefits, the Social Security

Administration will bill you monthly. If you do not receive cash benefits but enroll in Medicare Part B, HCFA will bill you quarterly.

Nonpayment of Premiums

Failure to pay your premiums could cause your coverage to be terminated. Medicare provides a 90-day grace period in which to pay premiums.

For premium Part A, entitlement will end on the last day of the third month after the billing month unless the beneficiary can show good cause for nonpayment and as long as the overdue premiums are paid within 90 days after the date entitlement would have been terminated.

For Part B, enrollment will end on the last day of the grace period, not to exceed 90 days after the month in which the premium is due. Payment of an overdue premium before the end of the grace period continues coverage without interruption.

If the beneficiary can show good cause for nonpayment within the grace period, an additional 90-day grace period may be granted. Good cause includes cases where the beneficiary was unable to make the payments due to physical or mental incapacity or because he believed payment had been made when actually it had not.

If you believe you will be unable to pay your premiums or you fail to pay your premiums, call your local Social Security office to explain why you have not paid. This will help establish the grace period and allow you time to pay without interruption of your coverage. Otherwise, your enrollment will be cancelled at the end of the grace period. Reinstatement at a later date will result in payment of a higher premium.

If you find you cannot pay your premiums due to low income, contact your local Social Security office or state Medicaid office to obtain information about qualification for Medicaid benefits, the Qualified Medicare Beneficiary program, or the Specified Low-income Medicare Beneficiary program. Medicaid will pay premiums for persons with income under 120 percent of the poverty line.

YOUR MEDICARE CARD

If you are already receiving Social Security or Railroad Retirement benefits, your Medicare card will be mailed to you when you are eligible for Medicare benefits. Figure 1-5 shows a sample Medicare card. If you must file an application for benefits, your card will be mailed to you after the application is processed and accepted.

Your Medicare card includes your name, your Medicare claim number (also called your Health Insurance Claim Number or HICN), your sex, information about your Medicare entitlement, and the effective date of your entitlement.

Figure 1-5: Sample Medicare Card

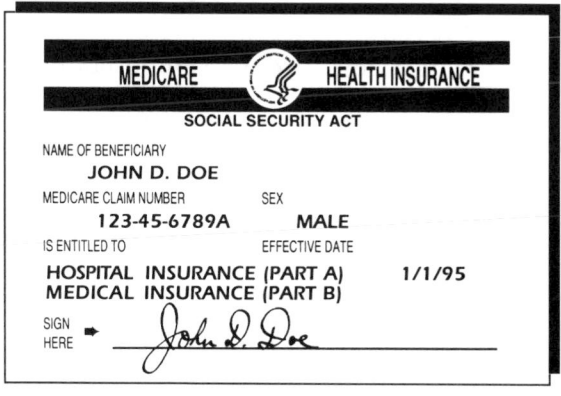

Your HICN provides information on the type of coverage you are entitled to and consists of your nine-digit Social Security number and either a number suffix, a letter suffix, a letter-number combination suffix, or a letter prefix. For beneficiaries who obtained coverage prior to 1964 through the Railroad Retirement Board, it is only six digits.

Special suffixes indicate that the beneficiary is entitled to Part A and/or Part B but not Social Security benefits, Part B benefits and premium Part A benefits, or Part B benefits only.

Your Medicare card is your "ticket" to coverage. It contains all the information needed to obtain Medicare-covered services. You should carry it with you at all times and show it when receiving medical or hospital services. Your doctor may ask to copy your card for his records; this is fine and should help eliminate errors related to your HICN and answer questions about your coverage or eligibility date. Also, be sure to sign your card immediately when you receive it.

It is important that, when corresponding with Medicare, you use your name and Medicare number exactly as they appear on your card. So, if there are any errors on your card, including the spelling of your name, your sex, or your entitlement, contact your local Social Security office for assistance in correcting the information. Once it is corrected and you are issued a new card, be sure to notify all physicians and other providers who might need this information.

If your card is lost, notify your local Social Security office or call the toll free number 1-800-772-1213 immediately. Someone there will help you file the correct information to obtain a replacement card.

Finally, *never* let someone else use your card. This includes your spouse or any other relative. Using a Medicare card to obtain payment for services provided to someone other than the person listed on the card is considered fraud and is punishable by fines and, possibly, imprisonment.

Preventing fraud is another reason it is important to let your local Social Security office know immediately when you discover your Medicare card is missing.

TERMINATION OF BENEFITS

Typically, benefits are terminated for one of two reasons: either nonpayment of premiums or death. Termination due to nonpayment of premiums takes effect at the end of the grace period (not to exceed 90 days). If premiums are paid during the grace period, no interruption in benefits will occur.

Should a person decide to terminate Medicare coverage, entitlement will end on the last day of the month following the month in which the written notice to terminate was received. Because beneficiaries face increased premium amounts for reinstatement of benefits, elective termination happens rarely.

CHAPTER 2

MEDICARE'S HOSPITAL INSURANCE

For many people, trying to determine which services and procedures Medicare will—and won't—pay for seems next to impossible.

The *concept* of coverage is fairly simple: according to Section 1862(a)(1) of the Social Security Act, Medicare covers items and services that are "reasonable and necessary for the diagnosis or treatment of an illness or injury, or to improve the functioning of a malformed body part." This includes a wide range of hospital, physician, and other institutional services.

Although there is no formal list of specific covered and noncovered procedures, supplies, or services, it is possible to ascertain from the law and the regulations which *categories* of services Medicare generally covers. It then becomes the challenge of the Health Care Financing Administration (HCFA) to get to the "nitty-gritty" regarding coverage. Through the many policy and procedure manuals, such as the *Medicare Intermediary Manual, Medicare Carrier's Manual,* and *Medicare Coverage Issues Manual,* HCFA provides guidelines that are more specific than the law about coverage of specific services.

This and the next chapter outline the types of services that are covered. This chapter discusses services covered under Part A of the law (hospital services) and the next chapter looks at services covered under Part B of the law (physician services).

COVERED PART A SERVICES

Generally, Medicare Part A provides coverage for the following services. (More information about each type of care is provided below.)

- *Inpatient hospital care:* care received upon admission to a hospital.

- *Inpatient care in a skilled nursing facility (SNF) following a hospital stay of at least 3 days:* care for patients who are recovering from an illness or injury and require skilled nursing services, i.e., more than assistance with daily activities of living.

- *Home health care:* care received in the patient's home.

- *Hospice care:* an alternative to hospital care for the terminally ill, providing pain relief, symptom management, and support services.

- *Blood.*

Benefit Period

Medicare measures a beneficiary's use of services under Part A by "benefit period"; there is a limit on how many days of hospital or SNF care that will be covered in each benefit period. A benefit period starts when a beneficiary is admitted to a hospital after Part A coverage begins. A benefit period usually ends when the beneficiary has been out of a hospital or other facility for 60 days in a row, including the day of discharge.

Part A coverage is renewed with each new benefit period. For each separate benefit period, the beneficiary must pay the inpatient hospital deductible ($736 in 1996). Note that this is different than standard health insurance which requires satisfaction of the deductible for a calendar year. To understand how a benefit period works, consider two examples:

Example 1: Mr. Happy entered the hospital on May 5 and was discharged on May 15; he used ten days of a benefit period. He was hospitalized again on November 20. Since more than 60 days passed between hospital stays, Mr. Happy begins a new benefit period for the second admission. Because it is a separate benefit period, Mr. Happy is required to pay the hospital deductible for the second stay.

Example 2: Mrs. Glum entered the hospital on January 15 and was discharged on January 20, using five days of a benefit period. She was readmitted to the hospital on February 3. Since fewer than 60 days passed between hospital stays, Medicare counts the first day of the second admission as day six of her benefit period. She does not begin a new benefit period until she has been out of the hospital (and SNF) for 60 consecutive days. Because the second stay is considered a continuation of the benefit period, she is not required to pay the hospital deductible for the second admission.

While Medicare does not place a limit on the number of benefit periods a beneficiary may accumulate over a lifetime, your out-of-pocket costs will begin to increase dramatically after 60 days in the hospital.

For a single benefit period, Medicare pays all charges (except the $736 deductible) for a hospital stay for the first 60 days of admission. After day 60, Medicare pays all charges except $184 per day through day 90. This charge of $184 per day will be billed to you by the hospital and is referred to as coinsurance.

If you require hospitalization beyond 90 days, you will be required to use "reserve days." Each beneficiary has a lifetime maximum of 60 hospital reserve days that can be used after day 90 of a single benefit period. Reserve days do not begin to accumulate again with a new benefit period.

For reserve days, you must pay coinsurance of $368 a day. If you are in the hospital longer than 150 days (90 days plus 60 reserve days), Medicare will no longer pay for hospital charges. To better understand how this works, consider our examples:

Example 1: Mr. Happy entered the hospital on May 5 and was discharged on May 15. He used 10 days of a benefit period. The only charge Mr. Happy is required to pay is the hospital deductible of $736.

Example 2: Mrs. Glum entered the hospital on January 15, was discharged on January 20, and was readmitted on February 3. She was discharged May 2; she was in the hospital for a total of 94 days. Mrs. Glum used the full 90 days of the benefit period plus four reserve days. According to the schedule, Mrs. Glum is required to pay the following:

First 60 days:	$ 736	(deductible)
Day 61-Day 90:	5,520	(30 days X $184/day)
Day 91-Day 94:	1,472	(4 days X $368/day)
Total:	$ 7,728	

Note that Mrs. Glum has only 56 reserve days remaining. For her next admission, she begins a new benefit period with up to 90 days coverage, as long as she is not admitted within 60 days of discharge. Were Mrs. Glum to be readmitted on June 30, which is fewer than 60 days from the date of discharge, the admission would be considered part of the previous benefit period and she would be required to use more of her reserve days at a cost of $368 per day.

You have a choice whether to use reserve days. If you decide not to use reserve days (possibly because you want to "save" them in case of catastrophic illness later or you just prefer not to use them), you will be responsible for all charges incurred. You must notify the hospital in writing of your decision when you are admitted or at any time up to 90 days after the date you are discharged. If you use reserve days and then decide you do not want to use them, you will have to request approval from the hospital. Contact the hospital's accounting department for help with this request.

All Medicare supplemental policies are required to pay for 365 days of care after all reserve days are used. Refer to Chapter Five for more information about supplemental policies and the services they cover.

Hospital Inpatient Care

Medicare Part A helps pay for inpatient hospital care if *each* of the following four conditions are met:

- A doctor prescribes inpatient hospital care for treatment of the illness or injury.

- The type of care required can be provided only in a hospital.

- The hospital participates in Medicare.

- The stay is not denied by a Peer Review Organization or a Medicare intermediary.

If a patient meets these conditions, Medicare will help pay for up to 90 days of medically necessary inpatient hospital care in each benefit period.

The major services covered under Part A for hospital inpatients are:

- Semiprivate room (two to four beds in a room).

- All meals, including special diets.

- Regular nursing services.

- Costs of special care units, such as intensive care or coronary care units.

- Drugs furnished by the hospital during the stay.

- Blood transfusions furnished by the hospital during the stay.

- Lab tests included in the hospital's bill.

- X-rays and other radiology services, including radiation therapy, billed by the hospital.

- Medical supplies, such as casts, surgical dressings, and splints.

- Use of appliances, such as a wheelchair.

- Operating and recovery room costs.

- Rehabilitation services, such as physical therapy, occupational therapy, and speech pathology services.

Personal convenience items, like a telephone or television in the room, private duty nurses, and extra charges for a private room (unless it is determined to be medically necessary) are not covered. If a private room or a television in the room is requested, and the hospital makes a charge for these items, the beneficiary will be required to pay the amount in addition to the deductible.

Remember that Part A pays for the hospital and its personnel and services, such as nurses, the room, etc. Part B will help pay for doctor's services, such as visits to the room, surgery, etc. In addition, any anesthesia received during an operation is payable by Part B, and will be billed separately from the doctor's services. Don't be surprised when you receive separate bills from the doctor, the anesthesiologist, and the hospital.

Note that you cannot submit bills to Medicare for your hospital stay; the hospital will submit the charges for you. Once Medicare has made a determination, the hospital will bill you directly for the deductible and any coinsurance amounts you owe.

Also, the hospital cannot require a deposit as a condition of admission to the hospital.

Inpatient Psychiatric Care

Part A helps pay for up to 190 days of inpatient care in a participating psychiatric hospital. This is a lifetime maximum; once Medicare has paid for 190 days, no more payment will be made. Benefit periods do not apply to inpatient care in a psychiatric hospital. However, most psychiatric care provided in a regular hospital is not subject to the 190-day lifetime maximum.

Notice of Noncoverage

The hospital must notify a patient *in writing* when inpatient care is no longer needed. This notification is called a notice of noncoverage (see Figure 2-1 below). If the patient disagrees with the decision and wants to remain in the hospital, the date and time the notice was received should be noted. Then, a written request for a review must be submitted to the state Peer Review Organization (PRO).

PROs are groups of practicing doctors and other health care professionals paid by the federal government to monitor the care given to Medicare patients. (They are discussed in more detail later in this chapter.) Such requests must be made immediately, because Medicare will cover the hospital stay for only two additional days after the receipt of the notice of noncoverage.

If the PRO approves the continued stay, Medicare will cover the additional days. If the PRO does not approve the continuation, the beneficiary will have to pay all hospital costs beginning on the third day after receipt of the notice of noncoverage.

Additional information about requesting a review for services denied on this basis is found in Chapter Six.

Figure 2-1: Sample Notice of Noncoverage

CONTINUED STAY DENIAL

DATE OF NOTICE:_____   BENEFICIARY:_____
ADMISSION DATE:_____   NAME:_____
HEALTH INS. NO.:_____   ADDRESS:_____
ATTENDING PHYSICIAN:_____   CITY,ST.,ZIP:_____

YOUR IMMEDIATE ATTENTION IS REQUIRED

Dear XXXXXXX:

MEDICAL CENTER has reviewed the medical services for "diagnosis" you have received from 00/00/00 through 00/00/00 and has determined that further hospitalization is not necessary. This determination is based upon MEDICAL CENTER's understanding and interpretation of Medicare coverage policies and guidelines.

FOUNDATION XYZ is the Peer Review Organization (PRO) authorized by the Medicare program to review inpatient hospital services provided to Medicare patients in this state. The PRO has concurred with our decision that beginning 00/00/00, further acute hospital care for "diagnosis" is medically unnecessary as it can be given safely in another setting. You will also receive a notice from the PRO confirming their decision.

We have advised your attending physician of the denial of payment for futher inpatient hospital care. You should discuss with your attending physician other arrangements for any further health care you may require. If you decide to stay in the hospital, you will be responsible for payment for all services provided to you by this hospital, except for those services for which you are eligible under Part B.

IF YOU DISAGREE WITH THIS DECISION: You may request by telephone or in writing an expedited reconsideration of the PRO's determination. An expedited reconsideration will be performed if you make your request while in the hospital. You should make this request immediately through the hospital or to the PRO at the address below.

IF YOU DO NOT REQUEST AN EXPEDITED RECONSIDERATION: You may still request a reconsideration. Instructions on how to request this reconsideration will be given to you in a notice sent by the PRO.

FOR RECONSIDERATION RESULTS: The PRO will send you a formal reconsideration determination of the medical necessity and appropriateness of your hospitalization and will inform you of your appeal rights.

IF THE PRO OVERTURNS ITS DECISION (i.e., determines that your care is covered by Medicare), you will be refunded any amount collected by the hospital except for payment of deductible, coinsurance, or any convenience services or items normally not covered by Medicare.

IF THE PRO UPHOLDS ITS DECISION (i.e., reaffirms that your care is not covered by Medicare) you are responsible for payment beginning 00/00/00.

Sincerely,

DOCTOR, M.D.
Chairman, Utilization Review

ACKNOWLEDGMENT OF RECEIPT OF NOTICE

This is to acknowledge that I received this notice of non coverage of services from MEDICAL CENTER on 00/00/00. I understand that my signature below does not indicate that I agree with the notice, only that I have received a copy of the notice.

Signature of beneficiary   Time   Date

Your Rights While You Are a Medicare Hospital Patient

Patients admitted to a Medicare-participating hospital receive a two-page document titled "An Important Message From Medicare, Your Rights While You Are A Medicare Hospital Patient." A copy of this message is provided in Figure 2-2.

This document explains patient rights in a Medicare-participating hospital and provides the name, address, and phone number of the state's PRO. This document also explains what to do if you think you are being asked to leave the hospital too soon (i.e., you receive a notice of noncoverage) and how to request a review when services are denied as noncovered.

All Medicare beneficiaries admitted to the hospital are given a copy of this message and are required to read and sign it. If you are admitted to the hospital and do not receive a copy, ask for one.

Inpatient Care in a Skilled Nursing Facility

A SNF is a specialized facility that offers skilled nursing care, or care that can only be performed by, or under the supervision of, licensed nursing personnel. Skilled nursing care differs from custodial care, which is help with activities of daily living, such as walking, getting in and out of bed, bathing, dressing, eating, and taking medication.

Custodial care can be provided by people without professional skills or training and is not paid for by Medicare. A SNF has trained, professional staff and equipment to provide skilled nursing care or skilled rehabilitation services and other related health services beyond those of daily living. Skilled rehabilitation services may include such

Figure 2-2: An Important Message From Medicare

An Important Message From Medicare
Your Rights While You Are A Medicare Hospital Patient

- You have the right to receive all the hospital care that is necessary for the proper diagnosis and treatment of your illness or injury. According to Federal law, your discharge date must be determined solely by your medical needs, not by "Diagnosis Related Groups" (DRGs) or Medicare payments.
- You have the right to be fully informed about decisions affecting your Medicare coverage and payment for your hospital stay and for any post-hospital services.
- You have the right to request a review by a Peer Review Organization (PRO) of any written *Notice of Noncoverage* that you receive from the hospital stating that Medicare will no longer pay for your hospital care. PROs are groups of doctors who are paid by the Federal Government to review medical necessity, appropriateness and quality of hospital treatment furnished to Medicare patients. The phone number and address of the PRO for your area are:

Talk To Your Doctor About Your Stay In The Hospital

You and your doctor know more about your condition and your health needs than anyone else. Decisions about your medical treatment should be made between you and your doctor. If you have any questions about your medical treatment, your need for continued hospital care, your discharge, or your need for possible post-hospital care, don't hesitate to ask your doctor. The hospital's patient representative or social worker will also help you with your questions and concerns about hospital services.

If You Think You Are Being Asked To Leave The Hospital Too Soon

- Ask a hospital representative for a written notice of explanation immediately, if you have not already received one. This notice is called a *Notice of Noncoverage*. You must have this *Notice of Noncoverage* if you wish to exercise your right to request a review by the PRO.
- The *Notice of Noncoverage* will state either that your doctor or the PRO agrees with the hospital's decision that Medicare will no longer pay for your hospital care.
  - If the hospital and your doctor agree, the PRO does not review your case before a *Notice of Noncoverage* is issued. But the PRO will respond to your request for a review of your *Notice of Noncoverage* and seek your opinion. You cannot be made to pay for your hospital care until the PRO makes its decision, if you request the review by noon of the first work day after you receive the *Notice of Noncoverage*.
  - If the hospital and your doctor disagree, the hospital may request the PRO to review your case. If it does make such a request, the hospital is required to send you a notice to that effect. In this situation the PRO must agree with the hospital or the hospital cannot issue a *Notice of Noncoverage*. You may request that the PRO reconsider your case after you receive a *Notice of Noncoverage*, but since the PRO has already reviewed your case once, you may have to pay for at least one day of hospital care before the PRO completes this reconsideration.

IF YOU DO NOT REQUEST A REVIEW, THE HOSPITAL MAY BILL YOU FOR ALL THE COSTS OF YOUR STAY BEGINNING WITH THE THIRD DAY AFTER YOU RECEIVE THE *NOTICE OF NONCOVERAGE*. THE HOSPITAL, HOWEVER, CANNOT CHARGE YOU FOR CARE UNLESS IT PROVIDES YOU WITH A *NOTICE OF NONCOVERAGE*.

things as physical therapy performed by, or under the supervision of, a professional physical therapist.

Medicare Part A helps pay for inpatient care in a SNF following a hospital stay of at least three days. The beneficiary's condition must require daily skilled nursing or skilled rehabilitation services, which can only be provided in a SNF, and the skilled care must be based on a doctor's orders. Medicare will help pay for care in a participating SNF if the patient meets the following five conditions:

- The condition requires daily skilled nursing or skilled rehabilitation services, which, as a practical matter, can only be provided in a SNF.

- The patient was in a hospital at least three days in a row (not counting the day of discharge) before being admitted to a participating SNF.

- The patient is admitted to the facility within a short time (generally 30 days) after leaving the hospital.

- The care in the SNF is for a condition that was treated in the hospital, or is for a condition that arose while the beneficiary was receiving care in the SNF.

- A medical professional certifies that the patient needs and receives skilled nursing or skilled rehabilitation services on a daily basis.

If the beneficiary meets these conditions, Medicare will help pay for a maximum of 100 days per benefit period of medically necessary care, but only if daily skilled nursing care or rehabilitation services are needed for that long.

If the beneficiary leaves the SNF and is readmitted because skilled nursing or rehabilitation services are needed for further treatment of a condition treated during the previous stay in the facility, and the readmission occurs within 30 days of discharge, a new three-day hospital stay is not required.

For each SNF benefit period, Medicare pays for all covered services for the first 20 days and the patient pays no deductible. For days 21-100, the beneficiary pays coinsurance of $92 per day; after day 100, the beneficiary is responsible for all charges.

As with inpatient hospital services, Medicare Part A is not responsible for paying for any physician services received in the SNF. Part B will pay for services provided in the SNF; the physician bills separately for his services. These are the major services covered under Part A for SNF inpatients:

- Semiprivate room (two to four beds in a room).

- All meals, including special diets.

- Regular nursing services.

- Physical, occupational, and speech therapy.

- Drugs furnished by the facility during the stay.

- Blood transfusions furnished by the facility during the stay.

- Medical supplies, such as casts and splints furnished by the facility.

- Use of appliances, such as a wheelchair, furnished by the facility.

Personal convenience items such as a telephone or a television in the room, private duty nurses, and extra charges for a private room (unless it is determined to be medically necessary) are not covered. Patients are required to pay for these items.

As with hospital services, the SNF submits charges to Medicare; patients do not file claims. The SNF will collect any coinsurance amounts due from the patient. Note that the SNF cannot require a deposit as a condition of admission to the facility unless it is clear that the services will not be covered by Medicare.

Notice of Noncoverage

As with hospital services, the SNF must notify patients *in writing* when they determine that skilled care is no longer needed. This notification is called a notice of noncoverage. If the patient disagrees with the decision and wants to remain in the SNF, the SNF must submit the claim to Medicare for an official determination.

The SNF cannot require payment until Medicare issues its determination. However, the facility can require the beneficiary to pay the coinsurance and for noncovered services while the claim is being processed.

Additional information about requesting a review for services denied on this basis is found in Chapter Six.

Home Health Care

A home health agency is a public or private agency that provides skilled nursing and other therapeutic services (such as physical therapy) in the beneficiary's home. Part A (and Part B) will pay for home health services furnished by a participating home health agency if the care is needed. To receive coverage for home health care under Part A, the following four conditions must be met:

- The care needed includes intermittent skilled nursing care, physical therapy, or speech therapy.

- The beneficiary is confined to the home.

- The beneficiary is under the care of a physician who determines the need for home health care and sets up a home health care plan.

- The home health agency providing the services participates in Medicare.

If you are unsure about whether you might qualify to receive this benefit, contact a local certified home health agency. They will review your case to determine if the services will be covered by Medicare.

The major services covered under Part A for home health care are:

- Part-time or intermittent skilled nursing care and home health aide services. (This can include up to eight hours of reasonable and necessary care per day for up to 21 consecutive days—or longer in certain circumstances).

- Physical, occupational, and speech therapy.

- Medical social services.

- Medical supplies.

Home health services *do not* include general household services such as doing laundry, preparing meals, shopping, or other home care services provided mainly to assist people in meeting personal, family, or domestic needs. Other home health services Medicare *does not* cover include:

- 24-hour-a-day nursing care at home.

- Drugs and biologicals (i.e., items needed to administer drugs, such as needles).

- Meals delivered to the home.

- Homemaker services.

- Blood transfusions.

The home health agency submits claims to Medicare; beneficiaries do not submit claims for these services. Medicare pays the full approved cost for all covered home health visits. Beneficiaries may be charged only for any services or costs that Medicare does not cover.

For durable medical equipment (like wheelchairs), the beneficiary is responsible for a 20 percent coinsurance payment for the equipment. Refer also to the next chapter on covered Part B services for more information about coverage of durable medical equipment.

Hospice Care

A hospice is a public agency or private organization that is primarily engaged in providing pain relief, symptom management, and supportive services to terminally ill people. It includes both home care and inpatient care, when needed, and a variety of services not otherwise covered under Medicare.

Under the Medicare hospice benefit, Medicare pays for a hospice to provide appropriate custodial care, including homemaker services and counseling.

Medicare Part A helps pay for hospice care if all three of the following conditions are met:

- A doctor certifies that the patient is terminally ill.

- The patient chooses to receive care from a hospice instead of receiving standard benefits for the terminal illness.

- Care is provided by a Medicare-participating hospice program.

Part A pays for two 90-day periods of care, followed by one 30-day period and, when necessary, an extension period of indefinite duration. A beneficiary may discontinue with the hospice during any benefit period, return to regular Medicare coverage, then later re-elect the hospice benefit if another benefit period is available.

There are no deductibles under the hospice benefit; the beneficiary pays only a small coinsurance amount for outpatient drugs and inpatient respite care. For drugs, the patient is responsible for five percent of the cost of the drug or $5 toward each prescription, whichever is less.

Under the hospice benefit, Medicare will pay for short-term inpatient respite care. This inpatient stay gives temporary relief to the person who regularly assists with home care. Each inpatient respite stay is limited to no more than five consecutive days. The patient pays five percent of the Medicare-allowed rate for this service, which amounts to about $5 per day, depending upon the area of the country.

Services covered by Part A when provided by a hospice include:

- Nursing services.

- Doctors' services.

- Drugs, including outpatient drugs for pain relief and symptom management.

- Physical therapy, occupational therapy, and speech-language pathology.

- Home health aide and homemaker services.

- Medical social services.

- Medical supplies and appliances.

- Short-term inpatient care, including respite care.

- Counseling.

The hospice benefit does not include payment for treatments other than for pain relief and symptom management of a terminal illness. However, treatments for other problems are usually covered under regular Medicare benefits.

Blood

Part A helps pay for blood, blood components, and the cost of blood processing and administration. "Blood" includes whole blood or units of packed red blood cells. For inpatients, Medicare will pay blood costs, except for nonreplacement fees (the amount some hospitals and SNFs charge for blood that is not replaced) for the first three pints. Referred to as the "blood deductible," beneficiaries are responsible for the costs of the first three pints of blood. The blood deductible is annual.

Patients can choose to pay nonreplacement fees, or they can arrange to have the blood replaced. Blood can be replaced by the patient (who donates his own blood) or arrangements can be made to have another person or organization replace the blood. A patient cannot be charged for any of the first three pints of blood that he replaced or arranged to have replaced.

Note that Medicare Part B also has a blood deductible. If you meet the blood deductible under Part B, you do not also have to meet it for Part A.

SERVICES PART A DOES NOT COVER

In addition to the specific noncovered services listed under each benefit category, Medicare also does not pay for the following:

• Custodial care.

• Care that is not medically reasonable and necessary.

- Care provided in conjunction with a noncovered service.

- Care not provided in the United States.

- Care not provided by a Medicare-participating hospital.

Custodial Care

Remember that custodial care is primarily help with activities of daily living, such as walking, getting in and out of bed, bathing, dressing, eating, and taking medication. Custodial care can be provided by people without professional skills or training and is often provided in a nursing home.

Medicare does not pay for nursing home or custodial care, even if supervised by a professional. (Under Part B, Medicare will pay for visits made by doctors to nursing home patients. See the next chapter.)

Care Not Medically Reasonable and Necessary

Medicare does not pay for services that it determines are not reasonable and necessary. This means that Part A will pay for services if the care needed could only be provided in the hospital.

If the care needed could have been provided on an outpatient basis, for example, or in the doctor's office, Medicare will not cover the inpatient services associated with the condition. If services are denied on this basis or admittance to a hospital is denied because Medicare determines that it is not medically reasonable or necessary, a review of this decision can be requested.

In the meantime, patients are responsible for payment of services not paid for under this exclusion.

Care Provided in Conjunction with Other Noncovered Services

This exclusion applies primarily to hospital inpatient services provided in conjunction with a noncovered service, such as plastic surgery. Medicare does not pay for cosmetic surgery (e.g., a facelift). If you require hospitalization as a result of an elective facelift, Medicare will not pay for the hospital or physician services associated with the procedure. The beneficiary will be required to pay for all services.

Care Not Provided in the U.S.

As a general rule, Medicare does not pay for services that are provided outside of the United States (which includes Puerto Rico, Guam, the Virgin Islands, and American Samoa). Three minor exceptions to this rule are:

1. If you are in the U.S. when an emergency occurs, and a Canadian or Mexican hospital is closer and provides the services you need, Medicare will cover the services.

2. If you live in the U.S. and a Mexican or Canadian hospital is closer to your home than the nearest U.S. hospital and provides the care you need, Medicare will cover the services (even if there is no emergency).

3. If you are traveling through Canada directly to Alaska from another state, or from Alaska directly

to another state, and an emergency arises, the care you receive at a Canadian hospital will be covered. Note that this does not apply if you are vacationing in Canada; you must be on your way to or from Alaska.

Care Not Provided by a Participating Hospital

While there are very few, some hospitals do not participate with Medicare. Should you require emergency care at a nonparticipating hospital, Medicare may cover the services. However, if it is not an emergency, Medicare will not pay for services provided at a nonparticipating hospital.

PEER REVIEW ORGANIZATIONS

PROs are groups of practicing doctors and other health care professionals paid by the federal government to monitor the care given to Medicare patients. Each state has a PRO that has authority to decide whether care given to Medicare patients:

- Is reasonable and necessary.

- Is provided in the most appropriate setting.

- Meets standards of quality generally accepted by the medical profession.

PROs work with hospitals and doctors to promote care that is most effective in treating illnesses and injuries. They also encourage quality care by distributing health care information and maintaining a toll-free telephone hotline to answer beneficiaries' health care questions.

PROs are responsible for reviewing beneficiary complaints about the quality of care provided by inpatient hospitals, hospital outpatient departments, hospital emergency rooms, skilled nursing facilities, home health agencies, and ambulatory surgical centers.

All complaints must be received in writing. If you cannot write your complaint, you can call the PRO and someone will take your information and write the complaint for you. You may have someone else submit the complaint for you (represent you), but you must give written permission to the representative.

The PRO investigates these complaints and renders decisions in writing. They will also tell you if you are responsible for payment when Medicare will not pay for a service. For a list of PROs in each state, refer to Appendix A in the back of the book.

CHAPTER 3

SUPPLEMENTAL MEDICAL INSURANCE

In the previous chapter you learned what types of services Medicare's Hospital Insurance, or Part A, covers. In this chapter you will learn what kinds of services are covered by Part B, Medicare's Supplemental Medical Insurance.

Medicare Part B covers physicians' and other practitioners' services and a wide range of "medical and other health services" not covered under Part A. Physicians' services include surgery, consultation, office and institutional calls, and services and supplies furnished incident to a physician's professional services. These services can be provided in an office, hospital, patient's home, or other facility, such as a nursing home, or on an outpatient basis.

In addition to discussing the types of services covered, this chapter also describes who can provide services and be covered under Part B. The Medicare program has expanded coverage for the types of practitioners who can provide services and receive payment for them. It is important to know this information; should you receive services from a physical therapist, for example, you will know whether Medicare will pay for those services.

COVERED PROVIDERS

Definition of a Physician

Medicare uses the term "physician" to include doctors of medicine (MD), doctors of osteopathy (DO), doctors of

dental surgery or dental medicine (DDS or DMD), chiropractors, doctors of podiatry or surgical chiropody, and
doctors of optometry. All physicians must be legally authorized (licensed) to practice by the state in which they perform procedures or services. Some doctors have a "limited
license" (see below) and so not all services provided by
them are covered.

Medicare will also reimburse for the services of auxiliary personnel: physician assistants, nurse practitioners,
clinical social workers, clinical psychologists, certified
registered nurse anesthetists, nurse midwives and physical
and occupational therapists. Information relating to payment
for these professionals' services, when provided incident to
a physician's services, is discussed in the following pages.

Practitioners other than MDs, DOs, and auxiliary personnel must meet certain standards and criteria for Medicare payment to be made. These conditions, and the services that are covered if provided by these practitioners, are
also described below.

Interns and Residents

For Medicare purposes, interns and residents are defined as physicians who are participating in an approved
postgraduate training program and physicians who are participating in a nonapproved program but who can practice
only in a hospital setting, e.g., a graduate of a foreign
medical school. Generally, the services of these physicians
are covered under Part A.

Regardless of the teaching program's approval status,
medical and surgical services performed by residents and
interns that are not related to their training program (e.g.,
that are performed while they are "moonlighting") and are
performed outside the facility where they have their training

program, are covered under the Part B program. Services performed outside the scope of their training program and in the emergency room or outpatient department of the hospital where they have their training program are covered under the Part B program as well. The intern or resident must be licensed to practice medicine by the state in which the services are performed.

Limited License Practitioners

Medicare also covers services provided by limited license practitioners (LLPs). While Medicare considers these practitioners physicians for purposes of payment, they are considered to have "limited license" because they are limited by their training and licensure to providing a certain type of services. LLPs covered by Medicare include dentists, oral surgeons, chiropractors, podiatrists and optometrists.

It is important to realize that even though these practitioners can provide covered services, not *all* services provided will be covered as determined by Medicare law. For example, Medicare law excludes payment for eye refractions regardless of who provides them.

Dentists

An individual with a DDS or DMD degree, who is licensed to practice dentistry and who is acting within the scope of this license when performing such services, qualifies as a physician under Medicare law. Services include any covered service that may also be legally performed by MDs and DOs.

Even though a dentist is considered a physician for Medicare payment purposes, Medicare law specifically excludes dental services from coverage *unless* the dental procedure is a necessary component of a larger procedure or service, such as treatment of oral infections. Therefore, just because a dentist is considered a physician does not mean regular services will be paid for by Medicare.

Oral Surgeons

Medicare covers services provided by oral surgeons just as it covers the services of dentists. Again, Medicare law excludes certain types of procedures from coverage, including most procedures related to the care of the teeth and supporting structures. Covered oral surgeons' services must be related to the care or treatment of an injury or illness, such as a jaw fracture.

Chiropractors

Coverage for chiropractic services extends only to treatment by manual manipulation of the spine to correct a subluxation demonstrated by X-ray (providing such treatment is legal in the state where it is performed). In addition to being licensed and legally authorized to provide services by the state in which the services are provided, a chiropractor must meet certain minimum educational and practice standards to receive reimbursement from Medicare.

Podiatrists

A podiatrist is an individual with any of the following degrees: doctor of podiatry (PodD or DP), doctor of surgical chiropody (DSC), doctor of podiatric medicine (DPM), or doctor of surgical podiatry (DSP), or who is a graduate in podiatry, master chiropodist, graduate chiropodist, or in a very few instances another podiatry degree. To be included as a physician under Medicare, the podiatrist must be licensed and may only receive reimbursement for services that are within the scope of his applicable state license.

Medicare will reimburse the podiatrist only for covered services performed; that is, treatment for flat foot is not a covered service so Medicare will not reimburse the podiatrist for treatment of this condition even if the podiatrist is authorized to furnish the treatment.

Optometrists

Effective April 1, 1987, doctors of optometry are considered physicians for Medicare purposes for all services they are authorized to perform under the laws in the state in which the services are performed. Medicare can help pay for cataract spectacles, contact lenses, or intraocular lenses provided by an optometrist following cataract surgery.

Nonphysician Assistants

Nonphysician assistants are personnel employed by physicians to provide auxiliary services. Medicare covers services provided by nonphysician practitioners, as long as the practitioner is supervised by a physician. In some cases, the services must be provided in a particular place to be covered. Medicare will cover services provided by:

1. *Physician assistants.*

2. *Nurse practitioners.*

3. *Certified registered nurse anesthetists and anesthesia assistants*, effective for services rendered on or after January 1, 1989.

4. *Independent qualified psychologists.* Diagnostic services performed by a qualified psychologist (who is not a clinical psychologist) whose practice is independent of an institution, agency, or physician's office, are covered if a physician orders such testing.

5. *Clinical psychologists.* The types of clinical psychologist's services covered by Medicare include:

   • Diagnostic and therapeutic services that the clinical psychologist is legally authorized to perform in accordance with state law and/or regulations.

   • Services and supplies furnished incident to a clinical psychologist's services if the requirements that apply to services incident to a physician's services are met. These services must be:

      — mental health services that are commonly furnished in physicians' offices;

      — an integral, although incidental, part of professional services performed by the clinical psychologist;

      — performed under the direct personal supervision of the clinical psychologist, i.e., the clinical psychologist must be physically present and immediately available;

— either furnished without charge or included in the clinical psychologist's bill.

6. *Nurse midwives.* A nurse midwife is a registered nurse who has successfully completed a program of study and clinical experience in nurse midwifery meeting guidelines prescribed by the U.S. Department of Health and Human Services (DHHS), or has been certified by an organization that is recognized by DHHS.

Coverage of nurse midwife services is limited to the maternity cycle (pregnancy, labor, birth, and the immediate postpartum period not exceeding six weeks). The services covered include those obstetrical and gynecological services furnished during the maternity cycle that would be covered if furnished by a physician.

7. *Clinical social workers.* Covered clinical social worker services include the diagnosis and treatment of mental illness. They do not include those services furnished to an inpatient of a hospital or skilled nursing facility (SNF) that the facility is required to provide as a condition for participation with Medicare.

8. *Independent physical therapists.* To receive payment under this provision, the therapist must be in independent practice. Medicare considers a therapist to be in independent practice if the therapist renders services free of the administrative and professional control of an employer, such as a physician, institution, agency, etc.; the patients treated are the therapist's own patients; and

the therapist has the right to collect fees for the services rendered.

The therapist need not be in full-time, private practice, but must be engaged in private practice on a regular basis, i.e., the therapist is recognized as a private practitioner and for that purpose has access to the necessary equipment to provide an adequate program of therapy. Also, to be covered the services must be performed in the therapist's office or the beneficiary's home. Services provided in a teaching institution are not covered since they are covered as part of the institution's services.

In addition to the qualifications of the therapist and the conditions for independent practice, the patient must be under the care of a physician and the services must be furnished under a written plan of treatment established by the physician or therapist caring for the patient.

9. *Independent occupational therapists.* For the services of the therapist to be covered, they must relate directly and specifically to a written treatment regimen established by a physician, after any needed consultation with the qualified therapist or by the occupational therapist providing the services. Also, the services must be reasonable and necessary (i.e., designed to improve function where an expectation exists that the therapy will result in a significant practical improvement in the individual's level of functioning within a reasonable period of time).

COVERED PART B SERVICES

The following is a list of Medicare Part B covered services. Each is described briefly in the following pages.

• Ambulatory surgical center services.

• Home health services, if not covered by Part A.

• Outpatient physical and occupational therapy and speech pathology services.

• Comprehensive outpatient rehabilitation facility services.

• Partial hospitalization for mental health treatment.

• Rural health clinic services.

• Federally qualified health center services.

• Laboratory services.

• Outpatient hospital services.

• Physicians' services:

— medical and surgical services, including anesthesia;

— commonly furnished supplies;

— services of nonphysician assistants, such as technicians, nurses, physical therapists and physician assistants;

— drugs and biologicals that cannot be self-administered;

— diagnostic tests;

— and radiology and pathology services.

• Durable medical equipment.

• Ambulance services.

• X-ray, radium, and radioactive isotope therapy, including materials and services of a technician.

• Surgical dressings and splints, casts, and other devices used for treatment of fractures and dislocations.

• Prosthetic devices that replace all or part of an internal body organ.

• Leg, arm, back, and neck braces and artificial legs, arms, and eyes.

• Therapeutic shoes.

• Screening pap smears.

- Screening mammographies.

- Flu, pneumonia, and hepatitis B vaccinations.

Ambulatory Surgical Center Services

An ambulatory surgical center (ASC) is defined as "a distinct entity that operates exclusively for the purpose of providing outpatient surgical services to patients, and has entered into an agreement with HCFA (the Health Care Financing Administration) to do so." In other words, it is a facility that provides surgical services that do not require hospitalization. Ambulatory means you can walk in and out.

Part B pays for the use of an ASC for certain approved surgical procedures as long as the ASC is participating with Medicare and is certified as an ASC. If you and your doctor determine that a necessary procedure can be performed at an approved ASC, Medicare Part B will pay for the use of the facility, the doctor's services, and any anesthesia services furnished in connection with the procedure(s) performed. Specifically included in the facility's payment are:

- Nursing services, services of technical personnel, and other related services.

- Use of ASC facilities.

- Diagnostic or therapeutic items and services (including simple preoperative lab tests, such as blood hemoglobin, urinalysis, or hematocrit).

- Drugs, biologicals, surgical dressings, supplies, splints, casts, appliances, and equipment.

- Administrative, recordkeeping, and housekeeping items and services.

- Blood, blood plasma, platelets, etc., except for those to which the blood deductible applies.

- Materials for anesthesia.

- Intraocular lens (IOL) implants.

Not included in the facility's payment are:

- Physician's services.

- The sale, lease, or rental of durable medical equipment to ASC patients for use in the patient's home.

- Orthotic and prosthetic devices.

- Ambulance services.

- Independent laboratory services.

Home Health Services

This benefit is the same as that available under Part A. If a beneficiary does not have Part A, he can receive home health services under Part B. If the beneficiary has both Part A and Part B, home health services will be covered under Part A.

Outpatient Physical and Occupational Therapy and Speech Pathology Services

Part B pays for physical and occupational therapy and speech pathology services if:

- The doctor prescribes the services.

- The doctor or therapist establishes a plan of treatment.

- The doctor periodically reviews the plan.

The patient may receive these services as an outpatient of a hospital or skilled nursing facility or from a home health agency, rehabilitation agency, or public health agency. Services can also be provided by an independently practicing physical or occupational therapist in the therapist's office or in the patient's home.

Medicare Part B will not pay for the services of an independently practicing speech pathologist. In all cases, the provider of services must be participating with Medicare.

Note that Medicare has established different payment rules depending upon what type of provider furnishes these services. If services are provided by the hospital, SNF, or other agency, the patient is responsible for paying any portion of the unpaid annual deductible plus 20 percent coinsurance. If the services are provided by an independently practicing therapist, Medicare will allow up to a maximum of $900 (in calendar year 1996). Medicare payment will be a maximum of $720, with the patient paying the remaining $180, plus any portion of the unpaid deductible.

Comprehensive Outpatient Rehabilitation Facility Services

A comprehensive outpatient rehabilitation facility (CORF) provides skilled rehabilitation and other services. Medicare will cover physicians' services, physical therapy, occupational therapy, speech therapy, respiratory therapy, counseling, and other similar types of services provided by a participating CORF. To be covered, your doctor must certify that the services are needed.

Medicare will also cover mental health services provided by a CORF. However, these services are subject to the outpatient mental health treatment limitation, which limits Medicare payment for mental health treatment services to 50 percent of the approved amount. This means that the patient is responsible for a 50 percent copayment, rather than a 20 percent copayment.

Partial Hospitalization for Mental Health Treatment

Also referred to as day treatment, Medicare provides coverage of outpatient mental health care when provided by a hospital outpatient department or community mental health center. Partial hospitalization services are not subject to the outpatient mental health treatment limitation.

Rural Health Clinic Services

Medicare Part B covers services of physicians, nurse practitioners, physician assistants, nurse midwives, clinical psychologists, and clinical social workers, as well as certain specified laboratory tests furnished by a rural health clinic. The clinic must be certified as a rural health clinic by HCFA for services to be covered.

Federally Qualified Health Center Services

Any Medicare beneficiary can seek services at a federally qualified health center, which may be located in urban or rural areas. As part of the federally qualified health center benefit, Part B will help pay for services provided by doctors, physician assistants, nurse practitioners, nurse midwives, clinical psychologists, and clinical social workers.

Certain preventive health services can also be covered. Under this benefit, you do not have to pay the annual deductible, but you will be responsible for the 20 percent coinsurance.

Laboratory Services

Unlike other benefits, Part B pays 100 percent of the charges for covered clinical diagnostic laboratory tests performed by certified labs that participate with Medicare. You do not have to pay any coinsurance for lab tests.

Laboratories can be independent, part of a hospital outpatient department, or in a doctor's office. Some laboratories are certified to perform only certain kinds of tests. A doctor should know whether the lab to which he is sending a test is certified to perform the test. If you have questions, talk to your doctor or you can contact your local carrier.

Outpatient Hospital Services

Services provided by a participating hospital to a patient on an outpatient basis are covered under Part B. This includes all types of services related to treating an illness or injury.

Physicians' Services

Physicians' services are the professional services rendered by a physician for a patient. They include diagnosis, therapy, surgery, consultation, and office, home, and institutional calls (visits).

Part B will cover physicians' services provided in almost any location, such as office, hospital, SNF, outpatient department, ASC, CORF, rural health clinic, patient's home, nursing home, etc.

A service may be considered a physician's service where the physician either examines the patient in person or is able to visualize some aspect of the patient's condition. Direct visualization would be possible by means of X-rays, EKG and EEG strips, tissue samples, etc.

Although most physicians' services are covered, Medicare does specify a few exceptions and impose a few conditions on this rule. Telephone calls between the patient (or the patient's guardian or representative) and the physician for the purpose of discussing test results, offering advice, etc., are not paid separately because they are considered part of the office visit or test performed.

Note also that the physician cannot bill the patient for this service just because Medicare will not pay for it. To do so is a violation of Medicare regulations.

Some practices have a policy of billing patients who fail to keep a scheduled appointment, known as a "no-show." *Under no circumstances* can patients be billed for a no-show; charging a Medicare patient for a no-show is considered fraud because no service was provided.

A visit to the doctor's office to obtain or renew a prescription, the need for which has been determined earlier, is not considered a covered service.

Medicare pays for consultations requested by the patient's attending physician and performed by a second physician or consultant for a patient. The consultation includes the history and examination of the patient as well as a written consultation report. Diagnostic tests ordered and performed by the consulting physician are also covered under Medicare.

Second opinions initiated by a Medicare patient are covered regardless of whether the procedure in question is covered. Medicare will pay for the history and exam of the patient and any diagnostic tests necessary for the physician to determine the necessity of the procedure in question. Third opinions will also be reimbursed if the original and second opinions differ.

Concurrent Care

In some cases a patient may require care by two doctors, or *concurrent care*. Medicare will pay for concurrent care if it is shown to be medically necessary. This means that the patient must present *different diagnoses* which require treatment by physicians in *different specialties*.

Consider the following: Mrs. Jackson has hypertension and diabetes for which she sees an internist. She suffers an acute myocardial infarction (heart attack) and must be admitted to the hospital. Once admitted, her attending physician calls in a cardiologist to perform a consult and then asks the cardiologist to treat the heart attack.

To be paid, each physician should report only the condition(s) (diagnoses) he is treating. In this example, the attending physician would report diabetes and hypertension while the cardiologist would report diagnoses related to the heart attack. In this way, the Medicare carrier will see that both physicians are treating separate problems (different diagnoses) so that the services of both doctors will be paid.

Charges for Filing Claim Forms

Charges to patients for filling out and filing their Medicare claim forms are not covered. Charging a patient for this service is a violation of the assignment agreement and the regulations (for unassigned claims). Patients are not liable for payment of this type of charge and the local Medicare carrier should be notified if a provider charges for completing and filing claim forms to Medicare.

Supplies

Supplies, such as gauze, bandages, etc., that are commonly furnished as part of the service are covered. The charge for the supply should be part of the charge for the service, or it should be provided without charge to the patient. The supply must also represent a cost to the physician for it to be covered. For example, if the physician gives an injection to a patient for which the patient provided the drug, the cost of the drug would not be covered as it represents no cost to the physician.

In some instances a practice can bill separately for supplies. The rule would apply for supplies a physician would not be expected to have in the office, such as crutches, or for services not considered medically appropriate to furnish in the office, including catheters and pessaries.

Services of Nonphysician Assistants

Nonphysician assistants are auxiliary personnel such as nurses, nonphysician anesthetists, psychologists, clinical social workers, physician assistants, technicians, physical therapists, and other aides. Direct personal supervision by the physician is required for any auxiliary personnel's services to be covered under Medicare.

This does not mean that the physician must be in the same room with the assistant. It does mean, however, that the physician must be *physically* present in the office suite and immediately available to help the assistant; the doctor cannot be on rounds in the hospital while the aide is providing a service.

Drugs and Biologicals That Cannot Be Self Administered

The term "drugs" refers here to medications prescribed by a physician. "Biologicals" are those items needed to administer the drug, such as needles, lances, and test strips used for blood glucose monitoring. Medicare will pay for a drug or biological if it cannot be self-administered, is provided incident to a physician's service, is approved, and is reasonable and necessary for the treatment for which it is used.

Let's consider two examples: Mrs. Peabody, who has arthritis, goes to her doctor's office for her monthly bursa injection. The drug used in the injection would be covered because Mrs. Peabody cannot administer this drug herself. Another patient, Mr. Mell, is diabetic and takes insulin. The insulin (the drug) and the needle and syringe (the biologicals) are not covered under this provision since Mr. Mell can inject the insulin himself. Note, however, that if the insulin is given to Mr. Mell by the physician or an aide in an emergency situation (e.g., diabetic coma), the drug and injection would be covered.

There are exceptions to this rule. Drugs that are covered under Part B include:

- Blood clotting factors given for hemophilia, even if they can be self-administered.

- Whole blood given to a hospital outpatient.

- Antigens prepared by the physician for a particular patient, which are given by or under the supervision of the physician.

- Immunosuppressive drugs given to a patient within 24 months after a covered organ transplant. (The time limit for coverage increases to 30 months in 1997 and 36 months in 1998.)

- Pneumococcal pneumonia and hepatitis B vaccinations.

- Epoetin alfa (EPO) provided to treat anemia in end stage renal disease (ESRD) patients or patients with chronic renal failure. (EPO is not covered when it is self-administered.)

- Injectable osteoporosis drugs given to a patient who has suffered a bone fracture as a result of post-menopausal osteoporosis, who cannot administer the drug herself, and who is confined to her home.

- Effective January 1, 1994, self-administered oral cancer drugs if they contain the same active ingredients as intravenously administered cancer drugs.

Diagnostic Tests

Among the types of covered diagnostic tests are:

- Laboratory services such as hematology and chemistry.

- Diagnostic X-rays.

- Isotope studies.

- EKGs.

- Pulmonary function studies.

- Thyroid function tests.

- Psychological tests.

- Basal metabolism readings.

- EEGs.

- Respiratory function tests.

- Cardiac evaluations.

- Allergy tests.

- Otologic evaluations (hearing tests).

These tests, including the materials and the services of technicians, are covered by Medicare as long as the tests are furnished by a physician or performed under his direct supervision.

Note that psychological tests performed by an independently practicing qualified psychologist are covered if they are ordered by a physician. Otologic evaluations are covered if they are performed by a qualified audiologist and are ordered by a physician to obtain additional information necessary to determine what type of medical or surgical treatment would be most beneficial to the patient.

For example, a test to measure a hearing deficit or to identify the reasons for the problem is covered if the test helps the physician determine whether surgery is warranted or not. However, testing performed to determine what type of hearing aid is necessary for the patient is not covered.

Radiology and Pathology Services

Included in this category are the performance and interpretation of X-ray and other types of radiological tests and treatments and pathology services, such as reading a specimen to determine if it is cancerous or not.

Durable Medical Equipment

Medicare covers the rental or purchase of durable medical equipment used in the patient's home. Repairs, maintenance, and delivery of this equipment, as well as supplies necessary to the use of the equipment, are also covered.

The equipment must be prescribed by a physician; equipment suppliers cannot send you equipment or solicit you to see if you want it. To be paid for by Medicare, your doctor must determine that you need the equipment and prescribe it for your particular condition.

As provided in the *Medicare Carriers Manual* and the *Intermediary Manual*, durable medical equipment is defined as equipment which:

- can withstand repeated use, i.e., could normally be rented and used by successive patients;

- is primarily and customarily used to serve a medical purpose;

- generally is not useful to a person in the absence of illness or injury; and

- is appropriate for use in a patient's home.

Items that are considered durable medical equipment include hospital beds, wheelchairs, hemodialysis equipment, iron lungs, respirators, intermittent positive pressure breathing machines, medical regulators, oxygen tents, crutches, canes, trapeze bars, walkers, inhalators, nebulizers, commodes, suction machines, traction equipment, and in some cases gel pads, pressure/water mattresses, and heat lamps.

Before you purchase or rent equipment, prosthetics, orthotics, or supplies from a durable medical equipment supplier, make sure the supplier is approved by Medicare and has a Medicare supplier number. Suppliers have to meet strict standards to qualify for a Medicare supplier number, and Medicare may not pay the claim if the supplier does not have a supplier number.

Suppliers are required by law to submit claims to Medicare on your behalf; they cannot charge you for this service. Claims are submitted to one of four regional carriers. These carriers and their addresses are included with the list of Medicare carriers by state shown in Appendix B.

Before payment for many items of durable medical equipment can be approved, Medicare requires the physician to complete a Certificate of Medical Necessity (CMN) form. This form helps the Medicare carrier determine that the equipment is necessary for treatment of the patient's condition.

Medicare allows some items of equipment to be rented, while others must be purchased. Some items may be either rented or purchased, or rented and then later purchased. The beneficiary is required to pay 20 percent coinsurance for the item. Medicare has developed a list of specific items of durable medical equipment and the conditions under which each item will be covered and paid. This list is provided in Appendix C. For more information about payment of durable medical equipment, refer to Chapter Four.

Ambulance Services

Expenses for ambulance services are covered under Part B when:

- the vehicle qualifies as an ambulance;

- the crew consists of at least two qualified members;

- the supplier certifies that its vehicle and crew meet the necessary requirements; and

- transportation in any other vehicle could endanger the patient's life.

Ambulance transportation can only be used to transport the patient to or from a hospital or SNF. Medicare will not pay for transportation to a doctor's office or to any other facility, such as an ASC or dialysis facility. Nor will Medicare pay for ambulance transportation because the beneficiary (or other person) thought it would be "easier" for the patient to travel this way; transportation by an ambulance must be required based on the patient's medical condition.

The ambulance transportation used must be local. If no local facilities in your area are equipped to provide the care needed, Medicare will cover transportation to the closest facility outside your local area that can provide the care you need. If you choose to go to another supplier when a local company is equipped to provide the care needed, Medicare will make payment based on the charge for transport to the closest facility.

X-Ray, Radium, and Radioactive Isotope Therapy

These services, including materials and the services of technicians, are covered provided they are performed under the direct personal supervision of a physician.

Surgical Dressings and Splints, Casts, and Other Devices Used for the Treatment of Fractures and Dislocations

Typically, surgical dressings are applied by the physician and are covered under the "incident to a physician's service" provision. However, if the dressing needs to be reapplied, by a family member for example, and must be obtained from a supplier such as a drugstore, it is covered under Part B.

To be considered a surgical dressing, the dressing must be applied to a lesion because of a surgical procedure performed by the physician. Items such as ace bandages, elastic stockings, foot coverings, knee supports, surgical leggings, and pressure garments are not covered as surgical dressings. Dressings required for other purposes, such as bedsores, are not covered.

Splints and casts are covered under Part B and must be provided as part of the treatment for fractures and dislocations. Splints and casts include dental splints.

Prosthetic Devices That Replace All or Part of an Internal Body Organ

Other than dental devices, prosthetic devices are covered by Medicare when they replace all or part of an internal body organ, including tissue, or replace all or part of the function of a permanently inoperative or malfunctioning internal body organ. Examples are cardiac pacemakers, prosthetic lenses, breast prostheses (including a surgical brassiere for postmastectomy patients), maxillofacial devices, devices that replace all or part of the ear or nose, and colostomy and ostomy bags and the necessary items required for attachment. A Foley catheter prescribed to a patient who has permanent urinary incontinence would be a prosthetic device.

Prosthetic lenses are covered when they are needed because of the patient's lack of the organic lens of the eye. Devices that could be included for coverage under this provision include prosthetic bifocal lenses in frames, prosthetic lenses in frames for far or near vision, and contact lenses worn in conjunction with lenses in frames prescribed for near vision. Tinted prosthetic lenses in frames (sunglasses) purchased in addition to regular framed lenses (nontinted lenses) are not covered because coverage is provided for the nontinted lenses.

Dentures are not covered. However, when a denture or a part of a denture is a built-in portion of a covered prosthesis, such as an obturator to fill an opening in the palate, the denture is covered as part of the prosthesis.

Supplies, repairs, adjustments, and replacement of prosthetic devices necessary for their effective use or due to wear or a change in the patient's condition, are covered when they are ordered by the physician.

Leg, Arm, Back, and Neck Braces and Artificial Legs, Arms, and Eyes

Braces include rigid and semi-rigid devices that are used to support a weak or deformed body member or to restrict or eliminate motion in a diseased or injured part of the body. This does not include elastic stockings and garter belts, for example. Special corsets, sacroiliac, sacrolumbar and dorsolumbar corsets, and belts are examples of covered back braces. Stump stockings and harnesses are also covered when they are essential to the effective use of an artificial limb.

Adjustments to these appliances are covered if the adjustment is required due to wear or by a change in the patient's condition, providing the adjustment is ordered by the physician.

Therapeutic Shoes

Medicare covers therapeutic shoes and shoe inserts for persons with severe diabetic foot disease. The doctor treating the diabetes must certify that the shoes are needed, and the shoes and inserts must be prescribed by a podiatrist (or other certified doctor) and supplied by a podiatrist, orthotist, prosthetist, or pedorthist.

Medicare limits coverage of therapeutic shoes to one pair of shoes per calendar year and needed inserts. Modifications to the shoes can be substituted for inserts. Payment for the shoes includes any charges for fitting.

Screening Pap Smears

Effective January 1, 1991, Medicare provides coverage of screening pap smears for women. Screening pap smears are those provided on a routine basis to all women, whether they have symptoms indicating the need for a pap smear or not. The screening smear is covered if the woman has not had a pap smear during the preceding three years or if she is considered at high risk of developing cervical cancer, which means that, based on the woman's medical history or other findings, her physician recommends she have the test performed more frequently than every three years.

Screening Mammographies

Beginning January 1, 1991, Medicare provides coverage of screening mammographies provided by a certified screening center. Payment is made based upon the woman's age and risk status. Also, depending upon her risk status, Medicare will pay for one test every 12 months or every 24 months. The age ranges, risk status, and coverage of the test are shown in Figure 3-1.

Figure 3-1: Conditions for Coverage of Screening Mammography

Age	Risk Status	Allowed Frequency of Test
35-39	All	One test
40-49	High Risk	One test annually
40-49	All	One test every two years
50-64	All	One test annually
65 & over	All	One test every two years

Flu, Pneumonia, and Hepatitis B Vaccinations

Vaccinations or inoculations usually are not covered unless they are directly related to the treatment of an injury, or the result of direct exposure to a disease or condition, such as an anti-rabies treatment or tetanus antitoxin or booster vaccination.

In the absence of injury or direct exposure, preventive immunizations against such diseases as smallpox, polio, diphtheria, etc., are not covered by the Medicare program. However pneumococcal, hepatitis B, and influenza virus vaccines are exceptions to this rule.

Medicare pays for pneumococcal pneumonia vaccine and its administration if it is ordered by a physician and the patient is at high risk for contracting this disease. Medicare will pay 100 percent of the cost of the vaccine and its administration; the beneficiary is not required to pay any coinsurance or deductible amounts for the vaccine. For unassigned claims, the beneficiary will be required to pay the difference between what Medicare actually paid and the amount billed by the physician.

The hepatitis B vaccine and its administration are covered when furnished to a Medicare beneficiary who is at high or intermediate risk of contracting hepatitis B and when ordered by a physician.

Effective for services provided on or after May 1, 1993, the influenza virus (flu) vaccine and its administration are covered when furnished in compliance with applicable state law. Typically these vaccines are administered once a year in the fall or winter.

For coverage purposes, Medicare does not require that the vaccine be ordered by a physician; the beneficiary may receive the vaccine upon request without a physician's order and without physician supervision. Medicare will pay 100 percent of the cost of the vaccine and its administration; the beneficiary is not required to pay any coinsurance or deductible amounts for the vaccine. For unassigned claims, the beneficiary will be required to pay the difference between what Medicare actually paid and the amount billed by the physician.

SERVICES PART B DOES NOT COVER

Medicare law specifically excludes certain types of services and procedures from coverage. However, just because Medicare does not pay for these services does not mean you cannot receive them.

For example, Ms. Taylor (a Medicare beneficiary) calls the local plastic surgeon because she has decided she wants a facelift. The doctor, upon discovering she is a Medicare beneficiary, explains to her that Medicare does not cover cosmetic surgery. He will, however, be happy to perform the facelift as long as she understands that she is responsible for the total charge. Ms. Taylor agrees to pay.

As another example, Mr. Thompson takes good care of himself, getting physical examinations every year, eating right, exercising, etc. The health insurance he has through his employer has never covered preventive care or routine physical exams. He is now a Medicare beneficiary and understands that Medicare does not pay for these types of services either. He still feels strongly that he needs annual exams and is willing to pay for them himself. His physician is happy to perform the exam and charge Mr. Thompson directly.

A doctor is not required (and should not) submit bills for noncovered services to the Medicare carrier. If you need Medicare to make a determination on the claim, possibly for your supplemental plan, the physician can send the claim to Medicare. Medicare will issue a denial notice and send a copy to you.

A list of excluded services together with a brief explanation of each is provided below.

Services Not Reasonable and Necessary

Medicare does not pay for services it decides are "not reasonable and necessary for the diagnosis or treatment of an illness or injury, or to improve the functioning of a malformed body member" (Section 1862(a)(1) of the Act). Medicare carriers use the following guidelines to make that determination. The procedure/service must be:

- Established as safe and effective.

- Consistent with the symptoms or diagnoses of the illness or injury under treatment.

- Necessary and consistent with generally accepted professional medical standards of care (i.e., not experimental or investigational or grossly inappropriate).

- Not furnished primarily for the convenience of the patient, the attending physician, or another physician or supplier.

- Furnished at the most appropriate level that can be provided safely and effectively to the patient.

Medical Necessity Denials

A medical necessity denial is one where payment for services is denied because they are determined by Medicare to be unnecessary or unreasonable for the diagnosis or treatment of the patient's problem. Other names for these types of denials are services that are not reasonable and necessary or medically unnecessary services. There are three basic reasons why services can be denied on this basis.

1. *The diagnosis does not "match" the service*, or the diagnosis does not really justify or make sense as a reason for the service provided. For example, a chest X-ray performed when the diagnosis was a fractured elbow would be denied for lack of medical necessity.

2. *Too many services provided in a short period of time*, such as more than one office visit per day or more than one nursing home visit per month. In these cases, the carrier questions the necessity for the intensity of the services provided.

3. *The diagnosis does not adequately justify the level of the service provided.* Called a level of service denial, this category involves either downcoding

(also known as a medical necessity reduction) or an outright denial. Most reductions occur with visits and consultations. For example, a patient visits the doctor because of a fever and sweats, for which the physician bills a Level V office visit (the highest level of office visit). In this case, the carrier is likely to reduce the level of service to Level II since it would seem more appropriate for treating this kind of problem. Alternatively, the service could be denied (rather than reduced) because the patient's problems do not justify such an intense level of service.

Note that many times, the services provided *are* actually necessary. But since carrier personnel are not medical personnel, they may not be aware of why the service provided was reasonable or necessary. For example, some carriers deny visual field tests when the diagnosis is migraine. Physicians understand that patients with migraines often experience field of vision problems, but the carrier's non-medical personnel (or computer) may not.

Also, many times the services denied on the basis of medical necessity are paid when the claim is appealed. As the example points out, the carrier could be wrong. The physician has the right to appeal the denial. With this appeal, he will need to provide further information to show why the service was needed. This could include further explanation about why the service is reasonable and necessary for the diagnosis; i.e., additional details about the patient's diagnosis that would explain why the tests or treatment were needed.

Medically unnecessary services have never been reimbursed by Medicare. They are a category of noncovered services, just as diagnostic X-rays are a category of covered services. However, the passage of the Omnibus Budget Reconciliation Act of 1986 (OBRA '86) included a requirement that doctors refund any amounts collected for services denied as not reasonable and necessary or that they not collect any amounts for services denied on this basis. Prior to this law, physicians could collect from the patient for these services, just as they still can today for other types of noncovered services. Congress, in enacting this new requirement, felt that since the services were not necessary, the patient should not have to pay for them. In addition, the law required the physician to "warn" the patient in advance that if a specific service was denied as not reasonable and necessary, the patient would be responsible for payment.

Please realize that while the intent of the law may have been to protect and help the beneficiaries, the implementation of the provision may not have worked as the law intended. Typically, the physician is much more qualified to make a determination about what types of services are needed by his patient than the carrier. With the carrier making the determination and the physician having to "protect" himself and warn his patient, physicians and patients can end up with an adversarial relationship rather than one of advocacy.

If the doctor has already collected money for the service, he is required to refund the money to the patient within 30 days. If the patient has made no payment, the physician cannot demand payment unless he notified the patient, in advance and in writing, that the service would not be covered and the patient agreed to pay.

Limitation of Liability Provision

The limitation of liability provision seeks to limit the liability for payment for services denied as not reasonable and necessary. There are two instances where this provision is invoked.

First, if neither the physician nor the patient knew, or could have been expected to know, that the service(s) would be considered not reasonable and necessary, the physician will be allowed to collect payment for that service.

Second, if the beneficiary knew, or could have been expected to know, that the service would not be covered, he is responsible for payment. However, it is unlikely that the patient would know the service would be denied if the physician did not know.

Who, then, is liable for payment? If the physician did not know, and the patient did not know that Medicare would deny the services as "not reasonable and necessary," the physician should be paid for the services. Under the limitation of liability, or waiver of liability, provision, Medicare will make payment for the service *once* if the physician and the beneficiary can show that they did not know that the service would be denied.

If, after Medicare accepts liability for payment, the physician submits a claim for the same type of service (for the same type of diagnosis), Medicare will determine that both the physician and the patient had knowledge that the services were medically unnecessary. The patient would be liable for payment (because he knew the services were not necessary).

Lack of knowledge, on the part of the physician and beneficiary, invokes the limitation of liability provision. The physician must prove that he had no reason to know that the service would be denied for lack of medical necessity. If the physician cannot prove that he did not know, and could not reasonably have been expected to know, that the services would be denied, he will be liable for the charges.

In other words, he cannot collect *any* money from the beneficiary.

Limitation of liability applies only to services denied as not reasonable and necessary. It does *not* apply to services denied as noncovered under any other section of the law. For example, a claim for a routine physical examination is not covered under general exclusions from coverage.

Consequently, limitation of liability does not apply and the patient is responsible for payment. The patient is always ultimately responsible for payment except in the case of medically unnecessary services.

The second exception to the rule applies if the patient was provided with a notice, prior to receiving the service, that explained that the service(s) could be denied as not reasonable and necessary. Physicians are exempted from making refunds or not collecting from the patient if they notified the patient in advance and the patient agreed to pay for the service. The law *requires* that the notice be in writing. The statement must include:

- a description of the procedure/service;

- the specific reason the physician believes the service will be denied;

- statement of the beneficiary's willingness to pay for the service, should it be denied; and

- the beneficiary's signature and the date signed.

A sample notice is shown in Figure 3-2. This form must be signed prior to receiving the services. The signed statement will be included in the patient's records.

Figure 3-2: Sample Advance Notice for Services Not Reasonable and Necessary

Medicare will only pay for services it determines to be reasonable and necessary under Section 1862(a)(1) of the Medicare law. If Medicare determines that a particular service, although it would otherwise be covered, is not reasonable and necessary under Medicare program standards, Medicare will deny payment for that service.

I believe that, in your case, Medicare is likely to deny payment for (specify and describe procedure(s)/service(s)): _____

_____

_____

for the following reasons (specify and describe all reasons physician believes service will be denied):_____

_____

_____

I have been notified by my physician that he believes that, in my case, Medicare is likely to deny payment for the services identified above, for the reasons stated above. I agree to be personally and fully responsible for payment should the services be denied.

Signature of Patient:_____
Date:_____

In situations where the same or similar services will be provided to the patient over a period of time, the doctor can ask you to sign a single notice *for that service(s) only.* Any other services provided where the physician suspects that Medicare may deny payment require a separate notice.

It is important to realize that, because Medicare decides that a service is not reasonable and necessary, it does not mean your physician is a "bad doctor" or that he is providing extra, unnecessary services just to get extra money from the Medicare program. Medicare carriers follow strict guidelines regarding utilization of services.

Sometimes, it is necessary for a patient to receive care that falls outside of these "standard" guidelines. Also, sometimes patients request services that Medicare has determined do not provide real benefits, such as Vitamin B_{12} injections. It is for situations such as these that this regulation exists.

If services you receive are denied as not reasonable and necessary and you do not fully understand the reasons, discuss the matter with your physician. He should be able to explain the medical necessity or the basis for Medicare's decision. Also, he may disagree with Medicare's decision and decide to appeal it. In either case, discussing the matter with you physician may alleviate some of your concerns.

Experimental or Not Approved by the FDA

Medicare does not pay for items that are considered experimental or that have not been approved for use by the U.S. Food and Drug Administration (FDA). Items must also be used for the purpose(s) approved by the FDA. In other words, if a procedure is approved for treatment of a particular illness and your physician wants to use it to treat a different problem, it is likely that Medicare will not pay since that use could be considered "experimental."

Nonphysician Services Not Provided Directly or Arranged for by the Hospital

Medicare excludes from coverage those services provided to a hospital inpatient by a nonphysician that were not provided directly by or arranged for by the hospital. Medicare law requires that services provided to hospital inpatients be provided by personnel under the direct employment of the hospital or by a supplier under contract with the hospital (usually to provide services not provided by the hospital).

If a supplier, such as a laboratory, provided a service to an inpatient but did not have a contract with the hospital to provide that service, Medicare would deny coverage. Also, services provided to hospital inpatients by hospital personnel or entities under contract with a hospital are covered under Part A. Services provided by authorized nonphysician assistants, such as PAs and nurse midwives, are covered services.

Services Related To and Required As a Result of Services Not Covered Under Medicare

Services provided in connection with other noncovered services (e.g., cosmetic surgery, routine examinations) are not covered by Medicare. For example, follow-up visits to a patient in the hospital who had cosmetic surgery would not be covered since the visits are provided in connection with a noncovered service.

Routine Services and Appliances

This category includes routine physical examinations (and any related tests, etc.); examinations of the eye for the purpose of prescribing, fitting, or changing eyeglasses; eye refractions; examinations for hearing aids; most immunizations; and eyeglasses, contact lenses, and hearing aids.

- Routine physical exams are those performed in the absence of an illness, symptom, complaint, or injury, or required by a third party, such as an insurance company, employer, government agency.

- In the case of eye exams, the purpose of the services, rather than the ultimate diagnosis, will be the criteria by which Medicare determines coverage for the services. In all cases, eye refractions are excluded from coverage.

- Vaccinations and immunizations, unless given for treatment or as a result of direct exposure, are not covered. The exception to this rule is vaccines for influenza virus (flu), pneumococcal pneumonia, and hepatitis B. For more information about this exception, refer to "Flu, Pneumonia, and Hepatitis B Vaccines" earlier in this chapter.

- Screening mammographies and pap smears, although they are routine and screening in nature, are exceptions to this exclusion. Refer to the information above under "Covered Part B Services" regarding these services.

Foot Care and Supportive Devices For Feet

Medicare specifically defines those instances in which foot care is excluded from coverage.

- Treatment of flat foot.

- Treatment of subluxation of the foot. However, for conditions such as osteoarthritis, bursitis (including bunion), tendinitis, etc., that result from or are associated with partial displacement of foot structures, Medicare will cover these services. Also, surgery to correct a subluxated foot structure that is an integral part of the treatment of a foot injury, or that is performed to improve the functioning of a foot or to alleviate a condition, is a covered service.

- Routine foot care, including cutting or removing corns or callouses, trimming of nails (including mycotic nails) and other hygienic and preventive maintenance. However, if the patient has a condition that results in severe circulatory problems or desensitization in the legs or feet, routine foot care could be covered. These illnesses and symptoms include, for example, diabetes mellitus, arteriosclerosis of the extremities, occlusive peripheral arteriosclerosis, Buerger's disease, chronic thrombophlebitis, and peripheral neuropathies involving the feet. In many cases, the patient must be under the active care of an MD or DO to be covered. Foot care otherwise considered routine can be covered if it is performed as an integral part of another covered service.

- Supportive devices for the feet. This includes orthopedic shoes and other such supportive devices. However, if the shoe is part of a leg brace, it will be reimbursed as part of the leg brace.

Custodial Care

Custodial care is care that is provided to assist the patient with activities of daily living. These types of services include help in walking, getting in or out of bed, bathing, dressing, feeding, using the toilet, preparation of special diets, and supervision of medication that can usually be self-administered. These not covered under Part B.

Personal Comfort Items

Items that do not contribute *meaningfully* to the treatment of the patient's problem are not covered by Medicare. Examples could include air conditioners, air purifiers, reclining chairs, etc.

Cosmetic Surgery

Cosmetic surgery is considered any procedure that is intended to improve appearance, such as a facelift. If, however, this type of surgery is performed to repair an injury, such as one resulting from a burn, the procedure(s) will generally be covered.

Services Rendered by Immediate Relatives or Members of Household

Medicare does not pay for services rendered by the patient's relatives or members of his own household.
This includes the:

- spouse;

- natural or adoptive parent, child, sibling;

- stepparent, stepchild, stepbrother, stepsister;

- father-in-law, mother-in-law, sister-in-law, brother-in-law, son-in-law, daughter-in-law;

- grandparent, grandchild; or

- spouse of grandparent or grandchild.

A member of the patient's household is considered anyone with whom the patient shares a common residence as part of a single family unit. Boarders and roomers would not meet the definition of a "member of the patient's household."

Dental Services

Medicare does not pay for items and services related to the care, treatment, filling, removal, or replacement of teeth or structures directly supporting the teeth. "Structures directly supporting the teeth" are the periodontium, which includes the gingivae, dentogingival junction, periodontal membrane, cementum, and alveolar process. Medicare may pay for these types of services if, for example, the procedure is part of the treatment for a patient who sustained a severe injury to the jaw.

Although dental services are excluded from coverage, certain services could be considered covered. If an otherwise noncovered procedure or service is rendered as an integral part of a covered service, the otherwise noncovered service will also be covered.

Examples include the reconstruction of a ridge as a result of and at the same time as the surgical removal of a tumor, wiring of teeth in connection with the treatment of a jaw fracture, extraction of teeth to prepare the jaw for radiation treatments of a neoplastic disease, and dental examinations prior to a kidney transplant.

Payment can also be made for services furnished incident to these services, providing the service is considered covered.

No Legal Obligation to Pay For or Provide Services

This exclusion applies to items and services furnished without an expectation of payment, for example, free immunizations. Note that fees waived for a given patient or class of patients, e.g., indigent or uninsured, do *not* meet the standard for no legal obligation to pay because, if the patient were not indigent or did have medical insurance, the physician would expect payment.

This exclusion applies where the physician or clinic is "giving away" an item or service, such as free screening tests, immunizations, etc., to *anyone* who wants it—no one is expected to pay for the service. In these cases, Medicare would not reimburse for services should a claim be submitted.

Services Furnished or Paid For by Government Instrumentalities

In general, this exclusion applies in three instances:

1. Services are furnished by a federal provider or agency, such as the Veteran's Administration (VA).

2. Services are furnished by a provider or physician at public expense pursuant to an authorization issued by a federal agency. This exclusion applies where a federal agency (e.g., the VA) requests a private physician to provide services for veterans for which the VA agrees to pay. In some cases, Medicare may pay secondary benefits. Services provided to Native Americans and their dependents under the Indian Health Service (IHS) Entitlement plan are

covered by Medicare with IHS as the secondary payer.

3. Services that have been or are expected to be paid for by a governmental entity. For example, services rendered to prisoners would not be covered under Medicare since the state would be responsible for their medical needs.

Persons eligible for CHAMPUS/CHAMPVA may be eligible to receive Medicare benefits as well. In these cases, CHAMPUS/CHAMPVA is secondary to Medicare. If, on the other hand, services are provided to an active member of the armed services in a civilian facility and it is expected that payment will be made by that branch, Medicare coverage does not apply.

Services Not Provided Within the United States

Medicare does not pay for services rendered outside of the United States. In some limited circumstances, coverage may be extended for certain inpatient hospital services and the associated physician and ambulance services provided in Canadian or Mexican hospitals. Services provided on board a ship may also be covered by Medicare.

Services Resulting From War

Items and services provided as a result of war or an act of war are not covered.

Services Paid or Expected To Be Paid Under Workers' Compensation

Medicare does not pay for services for which payment has been made, or can reasonably be expected to be made, under Worker's Compensation. This exclusion also applies to services for which payment has been made, or can reasonably be expected to be made, under an automobile, no-fault, or liability insurance policy or plan. For more information about coverage and payments in these situations, see Chapter Nine, "Medicare as Secondary Payer."

CHAPTER 4

PAYMENT OF MEDICARE SERVICES

Why is it important for beneficiaries to understand Medicare's payment methodologies? For two important reasons, first, understanding the "economics" of a system can help the user become a better consumer. A thorough understanding of how Medicare pays for services should provide you with needed information when interacting with hospitals, skilled nursing facilities (SNF), home health agencies, physicians, and suppliers.

Second, since the beneficiary is responsible for the hospital inpatient deductible, coinsurance for hospital and SNF stays, and a deductible and coinsurance for physician and other medical services, it will be very useful to understand how the payment system works so you will know how much you have to pay.

This chapter provides a somewhat detailed explanation of the payment methodologies used to pay for Medicare Part A and Part B services. Examples are provided at the end of each discussion to further illustrate how payment works.

In addition, a detailed explanation of the Explanation of Medicare Benefits (EOMB), the form Medicare sends you to explain the charges made for Part B services, how much Medicare paid, and how much you owe, is provided. This discussion should help you become more familiar with the form and the language used so you will be better able to read them.

PAYMENT UNDER PART A

Payment for Part A services requires very little involvement on the part of the beneficiary. Providers submit all claims and, unless the beneficiary has an extended stay in the hospital (more than 60 days), the beneficiary need only pay the inpatient deductible. This section provides an overview of Part A payment methodology with a focus on understanding the EOMB and determining how much is owed by the beneficiary.

What the Bill Looks Like

Hospitals and SNFs submit a form called a UB-92 to Medicare intermediaries. A copy of the form is reproduced in Figure 4-1.

In addition to the standard required information (e.g., patient name and address, identification number, account number, etc.), the UB-92 form includes space for reporting services provided and the charges made. Hospitals report "revenue codes," which are alphanumeric codes indicating the type of services provided. In addition, there is space to report special codes that indicate, for example, when Medicare is the secondary payer for the claim.

Understanding the Payment Methodology

To hold down the rapidly rising payments made by Medicare Part A, Medicare began paying for most inpatient hospital care under the Prospective Payment System (PPS) in September 1983. Under PPS, hospitals are paid a fixed amount for each Medicare discharge for inpatient services.

Figure 4-1: UB-92 Form

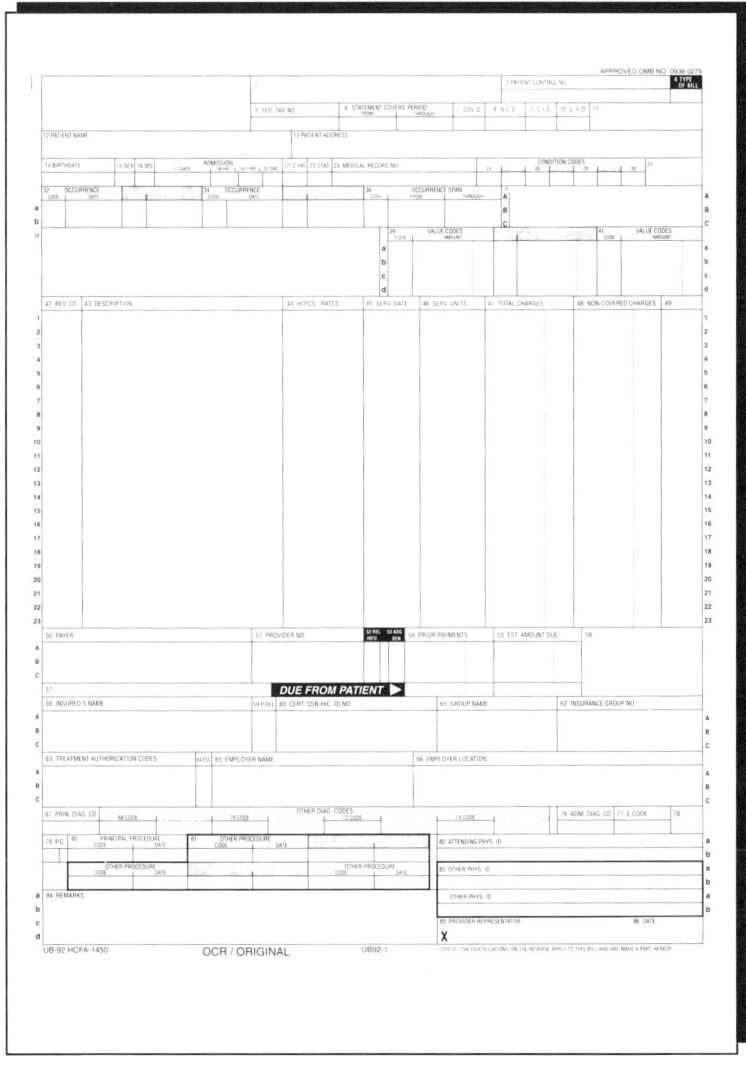

The fixed payment amount is based on the Diagnosis Related Group (DRG) into which the discharged patient is classified. Payment is not dependent upon the length of stay or the inpatient-related services provided during that stay; it is based solely on the patient's diagnosis at the time of discharge.

Diagnosis Related Groups (DRG)

A single DRG can be thought of as an "umbrella" diagnosis, such as chronic obstructive pulmonary disease (COPD). The groupings of illnesses or injuries that fall under each of the 495 DRGs are clinically coherent and relatively homogenous with respect to the resources used by the hospital to treat the patient's problem.

Because of this homogeneity, Medicare is able to make payments based on the DRG; each DRG has a set payment amount associated with it. If the payment is more than the hospital's costs, the hospital keeps the profit. If the payment is less than the hospital's cost, the hospital takes the loss.

The law requires the hospital to accept Medicare's payment as payment in full, regardless of whether the payment covered the costs. The patient is not responsible for differences between the hospital's costs and Medicare's payment. The patient pays only the applicable deductible and coinsurance amounts, plus any amounts due for non-covered items.

The DRG payment includes all services provided by the hospital to the inpatient. (For a more detailed list of covered items, see the discussion of covered inpatient services in Chapter Two.) Payment for items that are not covered by the Medicare program, such as a private room, are the responsibility of the patient. The patient will pay the difference between the cost of the covered item and the noncovered item. For example, if the cost of a semi-private room is $500 per day and the cost of a private room is $600, the beneficiary will be responsible for the difference, or $100 per day, for staying in a private room.

Payment for each DRG is roughly based on the expected costs and length of stay required on average to treat the diagnosis. Occasionally, costs for necessary care for a particular patient are unusually high or the length of stay is unusually long.

Since the hospital incurs extra costs for these special cases, it can receive additional payments to compensate for these extra costs. For a patient who has an unusually long stay compared to other patients in that DRG classification, the hospital is eligible to receive an extra payment called a "day outlier." For a patient whose treatment was extraordinarily more costly than other patients in that classification, the hospital can receive a "cost outlier" payment. The hospital must request these payments and substantiate its extra costs to receive the outlier payment.

Reasonable Cost

SNFs and home health agencies are exempt from PPS and are paid under the reasonable cost methodology. Some types of hospitals are also exempt from PPS and are also paid under the reasonable cost methodology. As the name implies, Medicare reimburses these facilities based on the costs incurred to treat Medicare patients. Institutions paid under this method must file cost reports to the intermediary; payment is then determined based on the costs allowed by Medicare (Medicare will not cover all costs incurred). Medicare payments are for aggregate services delivered during the year and, in general, are not allocated to individual patients.

Special exemptions to PPS apply to psychiatric and rehabilitation hospitals, psychiatric and rehabilitation units of acute care hospitals, pediatric hospitals, and long-term care hospitals. These hospitals are paid on a reasonable cost basis, subject to a ceiling on the rate of increase in inpatient costs.

Other types of hospitals are entitled to exceptions or adjustments to the payment made under PPS. These include:

- *Disproportionate share hospitals* — hospitals that serve a significantly disproportionate share of low-income patients — are paid an additional amount to cover the higher costs of treating these patients.

- *Sole community hospitals* — hospitals located in rural areas that are the sole source of care available to residents in that area — and small rural hospitals that are not designated as sole community hospitals have special payment rules.

- *Large teaching hospitals* receive additional payment to cover the indirect costs of teaching interns and residents.

ESRD Payment Methodology

Special payment rules have been developed for payment of services related to the treatment of end stage renal disease (ESRD) patients. Each dialysis facility receives a set payment amount per treatment, called the composite rate, which is the same whether treatment is furnished in the facility or in the patient's home. Medicare pays 80 percent of the composite rate, currently $139. The patient is responsible for any unpaid portion of the deductible and the 20 percent coinsurance.

The composite rate payment is considered full payment for all of the facility's costs related to each treatment, including all necessary dialysis services, equipment, and supplies, and routine physician's professional services. Direct patient care by the physician is not considered routine professional dialysis services and is billed to the carrier and paid in the same way as any other Medicare-covered physician's professional services. Certain laboratory services and drugs are not included in the composite rate either. Facilities also are paid $20 per session in addition to the composite rate for each self-dialysis and home dialysis training session provided.

Patients who dialyze at home choose between two methods of payment. Under Method I, the dialysis facility with which the home patient is associated assumes responsibility for providing all home dialysis equipment, supplies, and home support services. For this, the facility receives the same Medicare dialysis payment it would receive for an in-facility patient under the composite rate system. Under this arrangement, the beneficiary is responsible for paying any unmet portion of the Part B deductible and the 20 percent coinsurance on the Medicare rate to the facility. These claims are processed by the intermediary.

For Method II, called direct dealing, the beneficiary deals directly with a supplier of home dialysis equipment and supplies that is not a dialysis facility. There can be only one supplier per beneficiary and the supplier must accept assignment. The beneficiary is responsible for any unmet portion of the Part B deductible and the 20 percent coinsurance. These claims are processed by the carrier.

Understanding What Medicare Paid

When the Medicare intermediary has made a determination on a claim, the beneficiary receives a Medicare Benefit Notice which explains the determination. The Benefit Notice provides the beneficiary with information related to what services were paid for and in what amount as well as how much the beneficiary is expected to pay the provider (e.g., the hospital deductible).

From a beneficiary's standpoint, understanding payment for Part A services is relatively simple when compared to understanding payment for Part B services. The beneficiary's involvement in the process is limited to paying only the hospital inpatient deductible for hospital services and nothing for skilled nursing facility or home health services.

For those who have to be hospitalized for more than 60 days or whose stay in a SNF exceeds 20 days, the amount owed to the provider is calculated simply by multiplying the coinsurance amount per day times the number of days exceeding 60 or 20. In other words, payment is the same regardless of the covered services provided; no complicated 20 percent coinsurance amounts to calculate. It is for this reason that this section only briefly explains the Part A Benefit Notice.

A sample Part A Medicare Benefit Notice is shown in Figure 4-2. At the top you will note the intermediary's name and address and your health insurance claim number (Medicare number). The top of the form also informs you that this form is not a bill; it is for your reference and is sent by Medicare.

The back of the form contains an explanation of the information provided in the Notice. This information is printed on the back of all Notices.

Figure 4-2: Sample Medicare Benefit Notice for Part A Services (front)

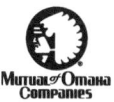

Contractor for

MEDICARE

MEDICARE BENEFIT NOTICE

Address reply to

MUTUAL OF OMAHA
Medicare Area
P.O. Box 1602
Omaha, Nebraska 68101

260107   DATE: 11/23/95

HEALTH INSURANCE CLAIM NUMBER

Always use this number
when writing about your claim

THIS IS NOT A BILL

This notice shows what benefits were used by you and the covered services not paid by Medicare for the period shown in item 1. See other side of this form for additional information which may apply to your claim.

1	SERVICES FURNISHED BY	DATE(S)	BENEFITS USED
	MEDICAL CENTER ATTN: ACCOUNTING KANSAS CITY MO 64131	10/16/95 THRU 11/02/95	17 INPATIENT HOSPITAL DAYS

2	PAYMENT STATUS

PAID DATE: 11/21/95
MEDICARE PAID ALL COVERED SERVICES EXCEPT:

    716.00 FOR INPATIENT DEDUCTIBLE.

IF NO-FAULT INSURANCE, LIABILITY INSURANCE, WORKERS' COMPENSATION,
DEPARTMENT OF VETERANS AFFAIRS, OR, IN SOME CASES, A GROUP HEALTH PLAN
FOR EMPLOYEES ALSO COVERS THESE SERVICES, A REFUND MAY BE DUE THE MEDICARE
PROGRAM. PLEASE CONTACT US IF YOU ARE COVERED BY ANY OF THESE SOURCES.
YOU DO NOT HAVE TO CONTACT US TO REPORT A MEDICARE SUPPLEMENTAL (MEDIGAP)
POLICY.

THE FLU SEASON IS HERE! PLEASE REMEMBER THAT MEDICARE NOW COVERS FLU SHOTS.

IF YOU WANT HELP WITH YOUR APPEAL

YOU CAN HAVE A FRIEND, LAWYER OR SOMEONE ELSE HELP YOU. SOME LAWYERS DO
NOT CHARGE UNLESS YOU WIN YOUR APPEAL. THERE ARE GROUPS, SUCH AS
LAWYER REFERRAL SERVICES, THAT CAN HELP YOU FIND A LAWYER. THERE ARE
ALSO GROUPS, SUCH AS LEGAL AIDE SERVICES, WHO WILL GIVE YOU FREE LEGAL
SERVICES IF YOU QUALIFY.

If you have any questions
about this record, call
or write

MUTUAL OF OMAHA MEDICARE
BOX 1602
OMAHA,   NE   68101-1602
TELEPHONE NUMBER   1-402-351-2860

FORM HCFA-1533 (9-83)

Figure 4-2 *continued*: Sample Medicare Benefit Notice for Part A Services (back)

EXPLANATION / GENERAL INFORMATION

A. **PAYMENT OF BENEFITS** – Payment for covered services was made on your behalf directly to the organization shown under **SERVICES FURNISHED BY** in item 1. Medicare paid for all services covered by the program except for items shown under **PAYMENT STATUS** in item 2. **YOUR MEDICARE HANDBOOK** tells you what hospital insurance pays for in a benefit period and what medical insurance pays for in each calendar year.

Hospital insurance covers inpatient hospital care, skilled nursing facility care and home health agency visits. Home health visits are also covered by Medicare under medical insurance, but the 2 benefits are handled separately.

Medicare medical insurance benefits for services you may have received from a physician or supplier are not ordinarily included on this record. If you have received physician or supplier services and the services are not mentioned under **PAYMENT STATUS** in item 2, a separate notice about these services is sent to you.

The number of covered days shown as used under **BENE-FITS USED** in item 1 represent only those used within the billing dates under **DATE(S).** If you received other covered services before or after the dates, separate notices about those benefits will be sent to you. A separate notice is sent each time payment for covered services is made on your behalf.

B. **SERVICES NOT PAID BY MEDICARE** – Medicare does not always pay the full cost of covered services in a benefit period. You are responsible for the specific deductible identified, if any, under **PAYMENT STATUS** in item 2 on the front of this notice. Deductibles must be met for each part of Medicare – hospital and medical insurance. A deductible applied to one part cannot be used to meet the requirements of the other. For a definition of "benefit period" and a detailed explanation of deductibles, see **YOUR MEDICARE HANDBOOK.**

Days still available in the benefit period or in the calendar year will not be paid for unless all Medicare requirements are met. The law does not cover all types and levels of institutional and home care. For a detailed explanation of Medicare requirements, see **YOUR MEDICARE HANDBOOK.**

Physician's services are not covered by Medicare hospital insurance, but they are covered by Medicare medical insurance. If you have the medical insurance and receive services in a hospital from a physician, Medicare pays for 80% of the approved charges for these services (if you have met the required deductible). You are responsible for the remaining 20%.

Hospital insurance never pays for services such as TV or telephone and private duty nursing. The added cost of a private room can be paid only if medically necessary. Medicare insurance never pays for some services such as meals delivered to the home and full-time nursing care. **YOUR MEDICARE HANDBOOK** describes these non-covered items in more detail.

C. **OTHER HEALTH INSURANCE** – If you have other health insurance that pays for some or all services not paid for by Medicare, you may use this notice to claim the other insurance benefits. Since the insurance company may keep this notice, make a record or copy before sending it to them. If a breakdown of billing charges is needed, you may obtain it from the facility shown under **SERVICES FURNISHED BY** in item 1.

D. **YOUR RIGHT TO RECONSIDERATION OF THIS MEDICARE BENEFIT DETERMINATION** – If you believe that Medicare should have covered more of your expenses, please ask the office shown just below item 2 for an explanation.

You may also request a reconsideration or review of the decision. The request must be made not later than 60 days from the receipt of this record for hospital insurance expenses or not later than 6 months from the date of issuance of this notice for medical expenses. The date of issuance appears on the other side of this notice in the upper right hand portion just above your **HEALTH INSURANCE CLAIM NUMBER.** The request should be sent to the office shown below item 2. If you are not satisfied with the reconsideration or review, you may request a hearing which must be made not later than 60 days from the receipt of the notice of reconsideration for hospital insurance expenses or not later than 6 months from the date shown on a notice of review for medical expenses.

IF YOU WANT HELP WITH YOUR APPEAL
You can have a friend, lawyer, or someone else help you. Some lawyers do not charge unless you win your appeal. There are groups, such as lawyer referral services, that can help you find a lawyer. There are also groups, such as legal aide services, who will give you free legal services if you qualify.

E. **FOR MORE INFORMATION** – If you have any questions not answered in **YOUR MEDICARE HAND-BOOK,** please call or write the office shown below item 2. The people there will be glad to help you. If you write, be sure to include your **HEALTH INSURANCE CLAIM NUMBER** exactly as it appears on this record.

Section 1

Section 1 identifies the facility that provided the services, the dates of service, and the number of benefit days used. The provider's name and address are found in the first column. Remember that a provider can include a hospital, skilled nursing facility, or home health agency.

The date or dates of service covered by the Benefit Notice are shown in the next column. The "Benefits Used" column indicates how many days of a benefit period were used. In our sample, the beneficiary was admitted on October 16, 1995, and discharged on November 2, 1995, which is a 17-day stay. This is reflected in the "Benefits Used" column.

Each Benefit Notice is "mutually exclusive," which means it pertains only to the single stay shown on the form. Previous or subsequent stays, whether within the same benefit period or not, will be reflected on a separate Benefit Notice. Previously-used benefit days will not be reflected in the Benefits Used column. Should you be hospitalized within 60 days preceding or following an admission, you will need to keep track of the total number of days used in a single benefit period. The hospital most likely will be keeping track as well.

Section 2

Section 2 contains information related to the payment status of the claim. In our sample, Medicare paid the hospital on November 21, 1995 and paid for all covered services. The beneficiary owes the hospital $716 (the 1995 deductible amount) for the hospital inpatient deductible. If, however, the beneficiary had stayed in the hospital for 67 days (until December 22, 1995), the Benefit Notice would have informed him that, in addition to the inpatient hospital deductible amount, he also owed coinsurance for seven days.

A reminder about appeal rights and where to obtain legal help is found at the bottom of the page. The name, address and phone number of the intermediary are found following this information.

Very many hospitals will check with the intermediary during your stay to see if you have previously satisfied the hospital deductible. If you have not, they will attempt to collect this amount and any other outstanding charges (for noncovered services) at the time of discharge. If you have a Medigap policy (supplemental insurance), the bill will be forwarded to that insurer, which will be responsible for payment of the deductible. Payment of charges for non-covered services will still be your responsibility, however.

Don't be afraid to take your time and check the bill over carefully before paying. Ask questions if there are changes you don't understand, whether you are unclear about what the item is or whether you question the amount being charged for the item. Hospitals do make mistakes in charging patients, so taking the time may save you some money.

EXAMPLES OF PART A PAYMENT

1. Mrs. Wilber was admitted to the hospital on May 10, 1996, for a scheduled hip replacement. The surgery went fine and Mrs. Wilber was discharged to a SNF on May 17. She stayed in the SNF for two weeks, until May 31. Mrs. Wilber used 7 hospital inpatient days and 15 SNF days. Charges for these services are calculated as follows:

Hospital stay 7 days $ 736 (deductible only)
SNF stay 15 days $ 0 (Medicare pays 100% for the first 20 days of a benefit period for a SNF)

Total owed $ 736

2. Mrs. Wilber is admitted to the hospital on July 15 because of breathing and other problems. She remains in the hospital for eight weeks, using 56 benefit days. However, since this admission is within 60 days of the previous admission, the first day of this admission is counted as day eight of the first benefit period. This means Mrs. Wilber does not have to meet the hospital inpatient deductible for this stay, but she will be required to pay coinsurance since the days used in the single benefit period totaled 63 days.

First 60 days   deductible met
Day 61-63 $ 552 ($184 per day x 3 days)

Total owed $ 552

3. Mr. Frances is very ill and is admitted to the hospital on January 12. He has many complicating illnesses, including diabetes, congestive heart failure, an ulcer, and high blood pressure. He remains in the hospital until April 29, for a total of 107 benefit days. When he returns home, he is cared for by a home health aide, who visits him every day until May 10. Mr. Frances will owe the following:

First 60 days: $ 736 (deductible only)
Day 61-day 90: $ 5,520 ($184 per day x 30 days)
Day 91-day 102: $ 4,416 ($368 per day x 12 days)
Home health care: $ 0 (Medicare pays 100% for
                                            home health care)

Total owed: $10,672

PAYMENT UNDER PART B

Payment for Part B services requires much more involvement on the part of the beneficiary than that for Part A services. Beneficiaries must understand what it means to participate and accept assignment, what it means when the physician is not participating, and how to determine the amount they must pay the physician or supplier. For these reasons, this section provides detailed information about the payment process for Part B services.

Medicare Fee Schedule and the Allowable Charge

Medicare pays for most Part B services using the Medicare Fee Schedule (MFS). It is derived by multiplying a national conversion factor, which is a dollar amount, by each procedure/service's relative value units, which reflect the resources involved in providing that procedure/service. Payment is adjusted based on the geographic area in which the procedure or service is provided. The MFS amount is also called the allowable amount that Medicare will pay.

The allowable is Medicare's full approved amount for a given procedure or service. When the Medicare carrier makes payment for the service, it pays 80 percent of the allowable to either the physician (under assignment) or the beneficiary (for unassigned claims).

Beneficiary's Copayment

Beneficiaries are responsible for paying the remaining 20 percent of the allowable, called coinsurance or copayment. Coinsurance for assigned claims is the amount, equal to 20 percent of the allowable, for which the beneficiary is responsible. For unassigned claims, the beneficiary is responsible for paying the difference between Medicare's 80 percent payment of the allowable and the physician's limiting charge.

Beneficiaries must also pay an annual deductible. The deductible is a set amount the beneficiary must pay each year before Medicare begins making payment for approved services. For 1996, the deductible is $100.

Physician Participation

Unlike Part A, providers under Part B are not required to participate with Medicare. Physicians and suppliers are allowed to choose on an annual basis whether or not to participate with Medicare. Agreeing to participate with Medicare means:

- The physician agrees to accept assignment for all Medicare claims he submits. Assignment, which is explained in more detail below, basically means the physician requests direct payment from Medicare.

- The physician agrees to accept Medicare's allowable as payment in full for the services, regardless of his actual charge.

Carriers publish two directories, the *Medicare Participating Physician Directory* and the *Medicare Participating Supplier Directory*, to help beneficiaries find participating physicians and suppliers. Beneficiaries can obtain a copy of either directory through the local Social Security office or from a local hospital. Carriers will also provide the directories.

Physician Nonparticipation

Electing not to participate with Medicare means the physician has the choice, on a claim-by-claim basis, to accept assignment. It does not mean the physician does not see Medicare patients or does not have to adhere to Medicare regulations. When the physician chooses not to accept assignment, the claim is considered to be unassigned. For unassigned claims, the physician must adhere to charge limitations, called limiting charges, determined by Medicare. Violation of the charge limitations is considered a violation of Medicare regulations.

The limiting charge is a limit or "cap" on the amount that nonparticipating physicians may balance bill beneficiaries. It is 115 percent of the nonparticipating MFS amount (and could also be called the nonparticipating allowable), which is 95 percent of the participating MFS amount. The limiting charge, then, is 9.25 percent higher (95 percent x 115 percent) than the allowable. If the allowable is $100, then the nonparticipating allowable is $95. This means the limiting charge is $109.25 ($95 x 1.15).

Assignment

Assignment is an agreement between the physician and the insured wherein the insured transfers his right to receive benefits to the physician; in return, the physician agrees to accept Medicare's allowable as payment in full for the services. Also, by accepting assignment the physician is requesting direct payment from Medicare.

There are some conditions of assignment to which the physician must adhere:

1. Under Medicare law, the physician *must attempt to collect* any unpaid portion of the deductible (this information is usually provided by the carrier) and the 20 percent coinsurance from the beneficiary.

According to the Office of the Inspector General, routine waiver of the deductible and coinsurance amounts is considered a violation of the law. This is because "it results in false claims, violations of the anti-kickback statute, and excessive utilization of items and services paid for by Medicare." In other words, a physician who routinely waives collection of the beneficiary's obligation is misstating his actual charge (thus causing Medicare to overpay). He is also considered to be giving the beneficiary a "bribe" to come to his practice (thus violating the anti-kickback statute), and inducing the patient to receive care that may not really be necessary (excessive utilization).

Many beneficiaries have supplemental insurance, which pays the deductible and coinsurance amounts. However, if the patient does not have this insurance, physicians are required to make a reasonable attempt to collect the coinsurance and the deductible from the beneficiary.

Medicare will consider attempts made by a practice to collect these amounts "reasonable" if the practice uses the same policy of collection for Medicare patients as it does for all other patients.

Two conditions may permit a practice to decide not to request payment for the coinsurance and deductible:

- *Hardship* — For those patients who are truly unable to pay the coinsurance and/or deductible (those who are indigent) and do not have supplemental insurance, collection of these amounts may be waived. Collection may be waived only to meet the special needs of a particular patient. All hardship cases should be fully documented.

- *An amount not cost effective to collect* — In cases where it would cost more to collect the payment than the amount being collected, a physician may decline to collect. For this exception to be valid, the physician should be able to identify, based on a cost analysis study, an amount below which collection is not cost effective for the practice.

Failure by a practice to attempt to collect the coinsurance and deductible is considered a violation of the regulations and the practice could be subject to penalties and sanctions. These sanctions include not only fines, but also possible exclusion from the Medicare program. Criminal charges may also be filed.

2. Under the terms of assignment, the physician is precluded from collecting, or attempting to collect,

more than the allowable charge. Note that the allowed charge is *not* the difference between the physician's charge and the amount Medicare pays, but the amount Medicare sets as the total allowable payment for the procedure or service. The following example illustrates this concept.

Physician's charge	= $1000
Medicare's allowable	= $ 900
Medicare pays 80% of the allowable	= $ 720
Physician collects 20% (coinsurance)	= $ 180

In this example, the physician's charge is $1000, but Medicare only allows $900, of which the program pays 80 percent, or $720. The patient pays only the difference between the *allowable* ($900) and the amount Medicare paid ($720), or $180. Under no circumstances may a physician who accepted assignment make a "side arrangement" with a patient to collect more than the allowable.

Regardless of the patient's willingness to pay more, it is still a violation and could cause the practice to be subject to sanctions and fines. *Any attempt to collect an amount above the allowable is a violation of the assignment agreement and should be reported to the carrier's fraud unit.*

3. Once an assigned claim is submitted to Medicare, the practice may not attempt to collect any amount from the patient until after the EOMB is received.

Any monies collected after the claim is submitted are likely to be an over collection and, as such, will be considered a violation of the assignment agreement. Practices are not, however, precluded from collecting the 20 percent coinsurance and any unpaid portion of the deductible from the patient at the time of service.

4. Medicare requires that all physicians, whether or not they participate, accept assignment for claims for the following types of services:

- Clinical diagnostic lab work performed in the office;

- Services provided to Medicare patients who are also Medicaid recipients;

- Ambulatory surgical center (ASC) services;

- Home dialysis supplies and equipment paid under Method II (direct dealing);

- Services provided by nonphysician practitioners, including physician assistants, nurse practitioners, clinical nurse specialists, nurse midwives, certified registered nurse anesthetists, clinical psychologists, and clinical social workers.

It is important to note that in 1994, over 92 percent of all claims processed by carriers were assigned. Of physicians, 72 percent were participating with Medicare. This means that many of the nonparticipating physicians submit assigned claims as well.

A Word About Accepting "Insurance Only"

Some physicians and clinics advertise that they will accept "insurance only." This means the physician or clinic agrees not to attempt to collect the coinsurance or deductible owed by the beneficiary; they accept Medicare's check for 80 percent of the allowable as payment in full. Be aware that this practice violates the terms of assignment and should be reported to your Medicare carrier.

Accepting "insurance only" is considered by Medicare to be a misrepresentation by the physician of his actual charge and so amounts to a "bribe" to induce patients to see the physician. If the physician's actual charge is same as the allowable amount, for example, $100, but he agrees to accept "insurance only," he really only expects to collect $80 for the service.

In this example, if the physician expects to collect only $80, that should be his actual charge, of which Medicare will pay 80 percent ($64) and you will owe 20 percent, or $16. By accepting insurance only, he has given you a discount of $4. Again, unless the physician is giving you a one-time break to help you out because you cannot pay, this practice is a violation of the terms of assignment and should be reported to your Medicare carrier.

What the Part B Bill Looks Like

Physicians submit charges on a form called the HCFA-1500 form. A copy of the form is reproduced in Figure 4-3.

Figure 4-3: HCFA-1500 Form

PLEASE
DO NOT
STAPLE
IN THIS
AREA

APPROVED OMB-0938-0008

PICA

HEALTH INSURANCE CLAIM FORM

PICA

1. MEDICARE (Medicare #) MEDICAID (Medicaid #) CHAMPUS (Sponsor's SSN) CHAMPVA (VA File #) GROUP HEALTH PLAN (SSN or ID) FECA BLK LUNG (SSN) OTHER (ID)

1a. INSURED'S I.D. NUMBER (FOR PROGRAM IN ITEM 1)

2. PATIENT'S NAME (Last Name, First Name, Middle Initial)

3. PATIENT'S BIRTH DATE MM DD YY SEX M F

4. INSURED'S NAME (Last Name, First Name, Middle Initial)

5. PATIENT'S ADDRESS (No., Street)

6. PATIENT RELATIONSHIP TO INSURED Self Spouse Child Other

7. INSURED'S ADDRESS (No., Street)

CITY STATE

8. PATIENT STATUS Single Married Other

CITY STATE

ZIP CODE TELEPHONE (Include Area Code) ( )

Employed Full-Time Student Part-Time Student

ZIP CODE TELEPHONE (Include Area Code) ( )

9. OTHER INSURED'S NAME (Last Name, First Name, Middle Initial)

10. IS PATIENT'S CONDITION RELATED TO:

11. INSURED'S POLICY GROUP OR FECA NUMBER

a. OTHER INSURED'S POLICY OR GROUP NUMBER

a. EMPLOYMENT? (CURRENT OR PREVIOUS) YES NO

a. INSURED'S DATE OF BIRTH MM DD YY SEX M F

b. OTHER INSURED'S DATE OF BIRTH MM DD YY SEX M F

b. AUTO ACCIDENT? PLACE (State) YES NO

b. EMPLOYER'S NAME OR SCHOOL NAME

c. EMPLOYER'S NAME OR SCHOOL

c. OTHER ACCIDENT? YES NO

c. INSURANCE PLAN NAME OR PROGRAM NAME

d. INSURANCE PLAN NAME OR PROGRAM NAME

10d. RESERVED FOR LOCAL USE

d. IS THERE ANOTHER HEALTH BENEFIT PLAN? YES NO *If yes, return to and complete item 9 a - d.*

READ BACK OF FORM BEFORE COMPLETING & SIGNING THIS FORM

12. PATIENT'S OR AUTHORIZED PERSON'S SIGNATURE I authorize the release of any medical or other information necessary to process this claim. I also request payment of government benefits either to myself or to the party who accepts asssignment below.

SIGNED DATE

13. INSURED'S OR AUTHORIZED PERSON'S SIGNATURE I authorize payment of medical benefits to the undersigned physician or supplier for services described below.

SIGNED

PATIENT INSURANCE INFORMATION

14. DATE OF CURRENT: MM DD YY ILLNESS (First symtom) OR INJURY (Accident) OR PREGNANCY (LMP)

15. IF PATIENT HAS HAD SAME OR SIMILAR ILLNESS. GIVE FIRST DATE MM DD YY

16. DATES PATIENT UNABLE TO WORK IN CURRENT OCCUPATION FROM MM DD YY TO MM DD YY

17. NAME OF REFERRING PHYSICIAN OR OTHER SOURCE

17a. I.D. NUMBER OF REFERRING PHYSICIAN

18. HOSPITALIZATION DATES RELATED TO CURRENT SERVICES FROM MM DD YY TO MM DD YY

19. RESERVED FOR LOCAL USE

20. OUTSIDE LAB? YES NO $ CHARGES

21. DIAGNOSIS OR NATURE OF ILLNESS OR INJURY. (RELATE ITEMS 1, 2, 3 OR 4 TO ITEM 24E BY LINE)

1. ___ . __ 3. ___ . __

2. ___ . __ 4. ___ . __

22. MEDICAID RESUBMISSION CODE ORIGINAL REF. NO.

23. PRIOR AUTHORIZATION NUMBER

24. A DATE(S) OF SERVICE FROM MM DD YY TO MM DD YY	B Place of Service	C Type of Service	D PROCEDURES, SERVICES, OR SUPPLIES (Explain Unusual Circumstances) CPT/HCPCS MODIFIER	E DIAGNOSIS CODE	F $ CHARGES	G DAYS OR UNITS	H EPSDT Family Plan	I EMG	J COB	K RESERVED FOR LOCAL USE

25. FEDERAL TAX I.D. NUMBER SSN EIN

26. PATIENT'S ACCOUNT NO.

27. ACCEPT ASSIGNMENT? (For gov't claims see back) YES NO

28. TOTAL CHARGE $

29. AMOUNT PAID $

30. BALANCE DUE $

31. SIGNATURE OF PHYSICIAN OR SUPPLIER INCLUDING DEGREES OR CREDENTIALS (I certify that the statements on the reverse apply to this bill and are made a part thereof.)

SIGNED DATE

32. NAME AND ADDRESS OF FACILITY WHERE SERVICES WERE RENDERED (If other than home or office)

33. PHYSICIAN'S, SUPPLIER'S BILLING NAME, ADDRESS, ZIP CODE & PHONE #

PIN# GRP#

PHYSICIAN OR SUPPLIER INFORMATION

(APPROVED BY AMA COUNCIL ON MEDICAL SERVICE 8/88)

PLEASE PRINT OR TYPE

FORM HCFA-1500 (U2) (12-90)
FORM OWCP-1500 FORM RRB-1500

Understanding the Payment Methodology

Physicians use standard coding systems to indicate the services and procedures they provide and the patient diagnoses. Procedures and services, including X-rays, lab work, anesthesia, diagnostic tests, office and hospital visits, consultations, and other services are coded using a system developed and maintained by the American Medical Association, called *Physician's Current Procedural Terminology*, or CPT.

Supplies and equipment are coded using a special coding system developed by HCFA, called *HCFA's Common Procedure Coding System*, or HCPCS.

Patient diagnoses, including illnesses, injuries, symptoms, and signs, are coded using a system developed by the World Health Organization and maintained by the National Center for Health Statistics, called the *International Classification of Diseases, Ninth Revision, Clinical Modification*, or ICD-9-CM. The ICD-9-CM codes appear in box 21 of the HCFA-1500 form, and CPT codes appear in box 24d.

After treating the patient, the physician completes the required information on the claim form and sends it to the carrier. The carrier processes the claim, renders a decision, and notifies both the physician and the beneficiary.

For assigned claims, the physician receives a check for 80 percent of the allowable charges and an explanation, called a remittance advice, of the charges approved for specific dates of services. The beneficiary receives an EOMB, similar to the one shown in Figure 4-9, which explains what services were paid for, who the provider was, and how much the beneficiary owes.

If the claim was unassigned, the physician receives a summary detailing what charges were approved and in what amount. The patient receives a check for 80 percent of the allowable amount plus an EOMB detailing what charges were approved and in what amount. The EOMB also indicates how much the patient owes the physician.

For assigned claims, the patient will owe 20 percent of the allowable amount for each approved service, after satisfying the deductible owed for the year. For unassigned claims, the patient will owe the difference between the allowable amount and the physician's actual charge up to the limiting charge (which is 115 percent of the allowable amount) for each approved service, after satisfying the deductible owed for the year.

Participating physicians can charge any amount they like for a service or procedure. However, they must accept Medicare's allowable as payment in full. Beneficiaries pay only the 20 percent coinsurance. If Dr. Friday submits a charge to Medicare for $1000 but the allowable is only $100, Medicare will issue a check for 80 percent of the allowable, or $80, and Dr. Friday can collect only the coinsurance from you, or $20. The difference between his charge and the Medicare payment amount is his concern.

For unassigned claims, nonparticipating physicians cannot collect more than the limiting charge amount from you, which is 115 percent of the nonparticipating fee schedule amount. If a nonparticipating physician accepts assignment, he cannot collect more than the 20 percent coinsurance. If a physician is nonparticipating and submits an unassigned claim for more than the limiting charge amount, he can be subject to fines and sanctions since this is a violation of Medicare law.

More About the Medicare Fee Schedule

The MFS is a fee schedule, which means it is a list of fees for each procedure or service provided by physicians. The fee schedule is based on a relative value scale, which "ranks" procedures and services on a scale based on their relative difficulty to each other. That is, since a heart bypass surgery requires more time and effort (resources) than removing a wart, the heart bypass will be higher on the scale than the wart removal.

Each procedure or service is ranked by assigning units of value, called relative value units (RVUs), to it. Procedures with more units are paid more than procedures with fewer units, since they are ranked higher on the scale.

The MFS considers three components when assigning values to each procedure or service:

1. the work required to perform it;

2. the practice costs associated with providing it; and

3. the malpractice expense associated with providing it.

The MFS also takes into consideration the geographic differences in practice costs (e.g., rent, labor costs, etc.) when calculating the total relative value units.

To arrive at a dollar amount for each procedure or service, the relative value units are multiplied by a national conversion factor, or multiplier, which is a dollar amount determined by Congress and provisions in the Social Security Act. Payment for assigned claims is calculated by paying either the physician's actual submitted charge or the fee schedule amount, whichever is lower. (Since the fee schedule amount is usually lower than the physician's actual charge, it is usually the allowable.)

Payment for nonparticipating physicians is a little more complicated, in part to encourage physicians to participate with Medicare. Assigned claims from nonparticipating physicians are paid at 95 percent of the fee schedule amount, called the nonparticipating fee schedule amount. For unassigned claims, the physician is allowed to collect the limiting charge, which is actually 115 percent of the nonparticipating fee schedule amount. The table in Figure 4-4 illustrates how payment is made.

While this may seem complicated (and sometimes it is), carriers provide a list of procedures and limiting charges for nonparticipating physicians to follow. For those ambitious persons who want to verify the charges made by their physicians, the MFS is published in the December 8, 1995, *Federal Register*. Fees for doctors in your area can also be obtained in the book *Does Your Doctor Charge Too Much?*, by Health Information Press (1-800-MED-SHOP).

For those who are not quite so ambitious, contact your local Medicare carrier if you believe that a physician has overcharged you. Also, your copy of the EOMB will provide this information and tell you how much you should pay.

If you do encounter a problem or question, don't overlook the simplest solution: speak directly to your physician or his insurance manager. They should be able to explain the discrepancy and help get it resolved. If your doctor has overcharged you, he is required to refund the difference between the limiting charge and the amount he charged. Should he fail to do this, call your carrier for help.

Figure 4-4: Payment for Physician Services

For this example, the Medicare Fee Schedule amount = $100

	Participating physician (All services assigned)	Nonparticipating physician (Assigned)	Nonparticipating physician (Unassigned)
Allowable charge	$100 (100% of MFS)	$95 (95% of MFS)	$95 (95% of MFS)
Beneficiary coinsurance	20% of allowable (.20 X $100 = $20)	20% of allowable (.20 X $95 = $19)	20% of allowable (.20 X $95 = $19)
Balance bill	Not applicable	Not applicable	15% of allowable (.15 X $95 = $14.25)
Total beneficiary out-of-pocket expense	Coinsurance $20	Coinsurance $19	Coinsurance + Balance Bill ($19 + $14.25 = $33.25)

Eight states have passed laws that further regulate the amount a nonparticipating physician can charge Medicare beneficiaries. The eight states and their specific laws are described in Figure 4-5. If you need more information, contact the state's insurance office or department of aging (phone numbers provided in Appendix D).

Billing Restrictions

Medicare (and other insurers) have policies Regarding how payment is made for different services. Understanding the details of how physicians' services are billed and paid will help you better understand your EOMB statements and the amount you owe the doctor.

Figure 4-5: State Laws Regulating Nonparticipating Physician Charges

Connecticut
Physicians are prohibited from attempting to collect more than the Medicare allowable charge from persons who qualify for the Connecticut Medicare Assignment Program (ConnMAP). To qualify for the ConnMAP program, the beneficiary's income must not exceed 165 percent of the qualifying income level established for entitlement to the ConnPACE program.

Massachusetts
Balance billing Medicare beneficiaries is prohibited. Physicians may not charge to, or collect from, a Medicare beneficiary any amount in excess of the Medicare allowable charge. This restriction applies also to ambulance suppliers. This restriction does not apply to suppliers of durable medical equipment.

Minnesota
Balance billing Medicare beneficiaries is prohibited. Physicians may not charge to, or collect from, a Medicare beneficiary any amount in excess of the Medicare allowable charge.

New York
Nonparticipating physicians are restricted to balance billing 105 percent of the nonparticipating physician fee schedule, which is 95 percent of the Medicare fee schedule. Multiplying 105 percent by 95 percent yeilds 99.75 percent. Effectively, nonparticipating physicians cannot collect more than the Medicare fee schedule.

Ohio
Balance billing Medicare beneficiaries is prohibited. Physicians may not charge to, or collect from, a Medicare beneficiary any amount in excess of the Medicare allowable charge.

Pennsylvania
Balance billing Medicare beneficiaries is prohibited. Physicians may not charge to, or collect from, a Medicare beneficiary any amount in excess of the Medicare allowable charge.

Rhode Island
Every physician must disclose to Medicare patients, in advance of treatment, whether the physician accepts Medicare assignment. Failure to make this disclosure (which can be accomplished by posting the information conspicuously in the office) shall not be allowed to balance bill the patient.

Global Surgical Charge

The global surgical charge is the charge made for a surgical procedure that can be thought of as a global package, or all-inclusive fee. The all-inclusive charge includes the surgery and some pre and postoperative care. Medicare has defined the elements included in the payment made for a surgical procedure.

For major surgeries, payment includes preoperative, intraoperative, and postoperative care.

• Preoperative care includes visits in or out of the hospital by the surgeon, beginning the day before surgery. Preoperative consultations and/or the initial encounter or evaluation is not included in the package.

• Intraoperative care includes all the usual surgical procedures, including all medical or surgical services related to complications that are considered part of the surgeon's care and do not require a return trip to the operating room.

• Postoperative care includes all visits, in or out of the hospital (or intensive care unit), within 90 days following surgery, and treatment by the surgeon of all conditions related to the diagnosis for which the surgery was performed.

Also included in postoperative care are miscellaneous services, such as dressing changes; local incisional care; removal of operative pack; removal of cutaneous sutures and staples, lines, wires, tubes, drains and splints; insertion, irrigation, and removal of urinary catheters, routine peripheral intravenous lines, nasogastric and rectal tubes; and changes and removal of tracheostomy tubes. Postsurgical pain management by the surgeon and supplies (other than those specified as separately payable) are included as well.

Any of the services or items listed above are considered to be part of the surgical package, which means that no additional charge should be made for them. The single surgical charge should account for the provision of the services/items in the above list.

There are some services that are not considered part of the surgical package, however, which means that, should they be provided, they may be paid separately. The charge for a major surgery does not include any of the following services:

• The initial evaluation(s) or consultation(s), even on the day of surgery.

• Diagnostic tests and procedures.

• During follow-up, treatment by the primary surgeon of conditions unrelated to the diagnosis for which the surgery was performed.

• Clearly distinct surgical procedures during the post-operative period which are not re-operations or treatment for complications.

• Medically necessary re-operations to correct complications.

- Services of other physicians, unless they are providing some portion of the surgical package.

- Immunosuppressive therapy for organ transplants.

- Supplies for services provided in a physician's office that are usually provided on an inpatient basis.

There are occasions when more than one physician provides services included in the global package (e.g., the physician who performs the surgical procedure may not furnish the follow-up care). Medicare pays the same amount for the package of surgical services whether the services are furnished by several physicians or only one physician. Each physician is paid directly for those services furnished by him. If part of the postoperative services are furnished by the surgeon and the remainder by another physician, then payment is based on a weighted percentage.

Global surgery payments for minor surgeries, nonincisional procedures, and endoscopy procedures performed through an existing body orifice include payment for:

- The visit on the day of the procedure, unless a documented, separately identifiable service is furnished (generally, for a problem different from that requiring surgery).

- The surgery itself.

- Postoperative care provided during ten days following the surgery.

Services related to treating the patient's underlying condition are not included in the package.

Multiple Procedures Reduction Rule

For multiple surgeries performed by the same physician on the same patient on the same day, Medicare allows separate payment for each procedure. Payment is made at 100 percent of the fee schedule amount for the highest valued procedure and 50 percent of the fee schedule amount for the second through fifth procedures. When more than five procedures are performed at once, the carrier will make the payment decision.

The beneficiary is responsible for coinsurance based on the reduced amount. Also, nonparticipating physicians cannot exceed the limiting charge for the *reduced* amount.

Assistant Surgeon

An assistant surgeon is a doctor who assists the primary surgeon in surgery. An assistant is not a PA or a nurse; it must be another physician. Medicare allows payment for an assistant surgeon for specified procedures. Payment is calculated at 16 percent of the allowable for the procedure. The beneficiary, then, will pay the coinsurance based on this reduced amount.

In some cases, it has been determined that an assistant is not needed and so Medicare will not make payment for one. Should your EOMB indicate that Medicare is denying payment for an unnecessary assistant, then you will not be liable for payment of the assistant. If there was a compelling medical reason for an assistant, then the claim should be appealed to see if the determination can be reversed. (See Chapter Six for more information.)

Bundled Services

Medicare has identified certain services, listed in Figure 4-6, which it considers to be included in an office, hospital, or other type of visit service. These are called "bundled services."

Figure 4-6: Bundled Services

Caloric vestibular test
Care plan oversight, over 60 minutes
Direction of advanced life support
Extra charges for:
  medical services provided after hours, at night, or at
    unusual hours
  non-office medical services
  office emergency care
  special supplies, patient educational materials, or group
    health education
  special reports or forms
  computer data analysis
Generation of automated data involving nuclear medicine
Optokinetic nystagmus
Physician phone consultation
Physician/team conference
Preparation of report
Prolonged services
Removal of sutures by the same surgeon
Special anesthesia services, including emergency anesthesia
  or anesthesia with hypothermia or hypotension
Specimen or device handling
Spontaneous or positional nystagmus study
Supply of a chemotherapy agent
Supply of a temporary tear duct plug, disposable endoscope
  sheath, paramagnetic contrast material, or surgical

Medicare will not allow separate payment for bundled services when they are performed incident to or in conjunction with another service even if the other service is performed on a different day. The physician may not attempt to collect from the patient or the patient's supplemental insurer for any of the identified bundled services. To do so is considered a violation of the limiting charge or of the assignment agreement.

Unbundled Services

In the CPT book, where applicable, codes are provided for components of procedures and a single code is provided for the "complete" procedure. The most common example is for a hysterectomy. There is one code to describe the complete hysterectomy and there are separate codes that describe each part of the hysterectomy (such as removal of tubes, removal of uterus, and removal of ovaries).

Under coding rules, complete procedures when performed are to be billed using the complete procedure code. Billing the components, called unbundling, is prohibited.

When procedures are unbundled, Medicare will "bundle" them back together and make payment for the complete procedure. Your EOMB will indicate when your physician has unbundled (usually unknowingly). The bundled procedure and the allowed charge will be shown also.

You are responsible for payment of the bundled code, not the component parts. Any attempts by the physician to collect additional amounts from you for the unbundled services should be reported to your carrier.

Site of Service Limitation

For physician services provided at least 50 percent of the time in the office setting, Medicare will reduce payment when the service is furnished in one of the following settings: hospital outpatient department, inpatient hospital, comprehensive outpatient rehabilitation facility, comprehensive inpatient rehabilitation facility, inpatient psychiatric facility, or emergency department.

The reduction, known as the site of service (SOS) limitation, applies if the procedure code is billed at least 50 percent of the time with office as the place of service. The rationale for applying this limitation is that, since the physician incurs less practice expense by providing the service in another location, the payment should be reduced to reflect the reduced resources used, and the additional payment made to the facility.

For procedure codes subject to the SOS limitation, the relative value units for practice expense are reduced by 50 percent when the service is furnished in one of the locations (other than office) listed above. The overall effect of the this is to reduce payment for the procedure or service by about 20 percent. The beneficiary's coinsurance responsibility is reduced as well; the beneficiary's portion is based on the reduced payment amount.

Supplies

Under Medicare regulations, payment for supplies is generally bundled into the payment amount for the surgical procedure performed. However, for certain specified surgical procedures performed in a physician's office, Medicare will make additional payment for the supply of a surgical tray.

If Medicare does allow payment for the surgical tray, the beneficiary is responsible for the applicable coinsurance. If Medicare does not allow payment for a supply, the beneficiary is not liable for payment of the supply *even if* he signed a notice in advance agreeing to pay. Physicians cannot require beneficiaries to pay for these items; to do so could be considered fraud or abuse.

Advance Notice for Elective Surgery

For unassigned claims, nonparticipating physicians must also notify the patient, in writing, prior to providing an elective surgery for which the charge is greater than $500. Elective surgery is defined as surgery that can be scheduled in advance, is not an emergency, and, if delayed, would not result in death or permanent impairment of health.

To be considered an emergency, the condition requiring surgery must meet the definition of emergency medical condition as defined in Section 1903(v)(3) of the Social Security Act. The Act defines emergency medical condition as ". . . a medical condition . . . manifesting itself by acute symptoms of sufficient severity (including severe pain) such that absence of immediate medical attention could reasonably be expected to result in (a) placing the patient's health in serious jeopardy, (b) serious impairment to bodily functions, or (c) serious dysfunction of any bodily organ or part." The notice for elective surgery must include:

- the fact that the surgery is elective;

- the physician's charge for the surgery;

- the approximate Medicare allowable;

- the amount by which the physician's charge exceeds the Medicare allowable; and

- the total out-of-pocket expense for which the patient is responsible.

Failure to provide this notification will force the physician to refund to the patient any amount collected above the allowable. Carriers are required to monitor adherence to this provision. To do so, they randomly sample surgery claims, contacting the physicians' offices who provided the surgery. A sample notice appears in Figure 4-7.

Purchased Diagnostic Services

In the past, it was common for physicians to bill patients and insurance carriers for diagnostic services that were procured or ordered on behalf of the patient but not actually provided by the ordering physician. Often, the ordering physician would "mark-up" the fee for the purchased service prior to billing. However, the Omnibus Budget Reconciliation Act of 1987 (OBRA '87) placed severe restrictions on this type of billing.

Effective March 1, 1988, physician practices are no longer allowed to mark up the cost of the test. In addition, the supplier's name, address, provider number, and net charge must be provided on the claim form.

Figure 4-7: Sample Advance Notice for Elective Surgery

I do not plan to accept assignment for your surgery. The law requires that where assignment is not taken and the charge is $500 or more, the following information must be provided prior to surgery. These estimates assume that you have already met the $100 annual Medicare Part B deductible.

Type of surgery: _____

Estimated charge for surgery $_____

Estimated Medicare payment $_____

Your estimated out-of-pocket expense $_____

Patient Signature:_____ Date:_____

ESRD Payment Methodology

As with facility services provided to these patients, Medicare pays for services provided by physicians to ESRD patients with a single payment amount, called the Monthly Capitation Payment or MCP.

MCP is a comprehensive monthly payment that covers all physicians' services associated with the continuous medical management of a maintenance dialysis patient. A separate MCP amount is determined for each locality and is used to reimburse all physicians in that area.

The monthly minimum is $132 and the maximum is $203. In addition, physicians can be paid $500 (subject to deductible and coinsurance) for providing self-dialysis training services for each patient under the physician's supervision during the training course.

Inpatient services provided by physicians can be paid under MCP or traditional fee-for-service under the Medicare Fee Schedule. Physicians cannot be paid both the MCP amount and fee-for-service. Physicians may also choose to be paid by the ESRD facility, which is paid an "add-on" payment for the physician's professional services. Administrative and certain other services are not included in the payment made to the facility.

Durable Medical Equipment Payment Rules

For payment purposes, Medicare classifies durable medical equipment into six categories. Each category and their payment options are discussed below.

Inexpensive or Routinely Purchased Durable Medical Equipment

Inexpensive equipment includes items costing less than $150. Routinely purchased equipment includes those items that are purchased (rather than rented) at least 75 percent of the time. Payment for these items is based on a fee schedule.

Also included in this category is used equipment, which Medicare defines as any equipment that has been purchased or rented by someone before the current purchase transaction and that has been used under circumstances where there has been no commercial transaction (e.g., equipment used for trial periods or as a demonstrator). Payment for these items is based on a fee schedule.

However, if a beneficiary rented a piece of brand new equipment and subsequently purchased it, the payment amount for the purchase should be high enough so that the total combined rental and purchase amounts at least equal the fee schedule amount for the purchase of comparable new equipment. For example, the fee schedule amount for a particular piece of equipment is $500 when the item is new, $375 when the item is used, and $50 per month when the item is rented. Mr. Jones rented the item when it was brand new for one month and then purchased it for $500. Medicare will allow $450 for the purchase ($500 purchase price less $50 for one month's rental), rather than $375.

Items Requiring Frequent and Substantial Servicing

For items identified as requiring frequent or substantial servicing, Medicare will pay for rented items only. Payment is based on a fee schedule.

Customized Items

Customized items are those that have been specially made or modified for an individual patient. Payment determinations are made based on each item by the individual carrier.

Other Prosthetic and Orthotic Devices

This category includes all prosthetic and orthotic devices except: items requiring frequent and substantial servicing; certain customized items; transcutaneous electrical nerve stimulators; parenteral/enteral nutritional supplies and equipment; and intraocular lenses. Payment is made based on a fee schedule for purchased items only.

Capped Rental Items

This is equipment for which the rental amount is "capped" or limited. Payment is made in one of three ways: (1) on a monthly rental basis, not to exceed a period of continuous use of 15 months; (2) on a purchase option basis not to exceed a period of continuous use of 13 months; or (3) on a purchase basis for some specified items.

Rental payments may not exceed a period of continuous use of longer than 15 months. After 15 months of rent have been paid, the supplier must continue to provide the item without charge, other than for maintenance and servicing fees, until medical necessity ends or Medicare coverage ceases (e.g., patient enrolls in an HMO).

Unless there is a break in the patient's need for the item of at least 60 days, medical necessity is presumed to continue. Medicare will also pay to replace an item after it has exhausted its useful lifetime (which is not less than five years from the date of delivery to the beneficiary) or if the item is lost or irreparably damaged.

Effective May 1, 1991, suppliers must give beneficiaries the option of converting their rental equipment to purchased equipment during their tenth continuous rental month. The supplier must notify the carrier that it has contacted the beneficiary and furnished him with the option of either purchase or continued rental. The beneficiary has one month from the date the supplier makes the offer to accept this option.

If purchase is declined, rental payments will be continued until the 15th month. If purchase is chosen, the carrier will continue to make rental payments until a total of 13 payments have been made. At that time, Medicare payment will cease and the supplier must transfer title to the equipment to the beneficiary.

Also effective May 1, 1991, suppliers must give beneficiaries entitled to electric wheelchairs the option of purchasing them at the time the wheelchair is furnished. The supplier must notify the carrier that the beneficiary has been advised of the purchase option. If the beneficiary chooses to purchase, Medicare will make payment based on a fee schedule. If the beneficiary chooses to rent, Medicare will make payment for 15 continuous months of rental. The beneficiary will again be given the option of purchasing the wheelchair in the tenth month of rental, as discussed above.

Oxygen and Oxygen Equipment

This includes stationary and portable oxygen equipment and the oxygen itself. These items are paid based on a monthly rate per beneficiary. Purchased equipment is not covered.

Other Charges

Suppliers of durable medical equipment may make additional charges other than those that cover the equipment and supplies themselves. Delivery and service charges are included in the payment for the equipment; they are not payable separately unless the supplier incurs "extraordinary expense."

For example, Medicare will cover all reasonable and necessary expenses incurred in the installation of home dialysis equipment, but not those expenses attributable to items that are basically for the purpose of improving the patient's home, such as plumbing or electrical work beyond that necessary to tie in with existing power or water lines. Delivery and installation charges are allowed for dialysis equipment because testing of the equipment is involved.

Medicare will also pay for interest and carrying charges for dialysis equipment if all of the following conditions are met:

- the interest and/or carrying charge is separately identified on the claim;

- it is the usual and acceptable practice in the area for suppliers to make such an extra charge;

- the practice of making an extra charge applies to all purchasers; and

- the additional amount charged is no higher than the applicable state or local government interest limit.

However, penalty charges assessed because of failure to make payments on time are not covered under Medicare. The supplier (or physician) may collect this amount from the beneficiary.

Additional expenses for deluxe features or items chosen for aesthetic reasons or added convenience do not meet the "reasonable and necessary" test for coverage. Thus, where a service or item is medically necessary and covered under the Medicare program, and the patient wishes to obtain extra or deluxe features, payment is made based upon the payment amount for the kind of item or service normally used to meet the intended purpose (i.e., the standard item). Medically necessary extra features, such as a power-operated wheelchair for a patient who is not strong enough to operate a manual wheelchair, are payable.

Time Limits for Submitting Claims

Medicare imposes a time limit for filing claims for Part B services. If claims are not filed within the specified time limit, Medicare will not make payment on the claim and the beneficiary can be held responsible only for payment of the applicable coinsurance and unpaid deductible.

Since September 1, 1990, all providers, whether participating or nonparticipating, have been required to submit Part B Medicare claims on behalf of the beneficiary. Providers are not allowed to charge the beneficiary for this service. All Medicare claims must be filed by the end of the year following the year in which the service was rendered, except for services rendered in the last three months of the year, which can be counted as being provided in the next year. For example:

Services Provided Between:	*Must Be Submitted By:*
Jan. 1 - Sept. 30, 1995	Dec. 31, 1996
Oct. 1 - Sept. 30, 1996	Dec. 31, 1997
Oct. 1 - Sept. 30, 1997	Dec. 31, 1998

Note that this requirement was amended in 1994 such that assigned claims not submitted within *one year of the date of service* will have payment reduced by ten percent. Beneficiaries are not responsible for the payment reduction; you are required to pay the coinsurance based on the reduced payment amount.

Similarly, if any claim is not submitted within the time limit as outlined above, the carrier will deny payment in full. The beneficiary is not responsible for payment of the full allowable but is responsible for payment of the coinsurance that would have been required had the claim been paid and any unpaid deductible amount. The physician loses the remaining payment of the allowable.

Beneficiaries who have other insurance that is required to pay benefits before Medicare pays can submit these claims themselves; physicians are not required to submit these claims to the primary insurer (although many do if they are accepting assignment). Physicians are required to submit claims only for Medicare covered services. Claims for noncovered services are typically not submitted to Medicare and payment for the services is the beneficiary's responsibility.

However, some beneficiaries have supplemental insurance that pays for items and services not paid for by Medicare, such as preventive care or care provided outside the United States. These Medigap plans usually require a copy of Medicare's denial before making payment, so these claims should be submitted by the physician even the services are not covered by Medicare.

Time Limits for Paying Claims

Just as physicians have time limits for filing claims, Medicare carriers have limits on how long they can take to process and pay a claim. Since 1987, carriers have been required to follow prompt payment standards, which are shown in Figure 4-8.

Note that in 1994, the regulation was changed to encourage submission of electronic claims (sending claims via computer rather than printed on paper). Starting in that year, you can see that there is no differential for participating versus nonparticipating physicians; the difference is based on the type of submission.

Figure 4-8: Time Limits for Processing Claims

Year	Participating Physicians	Nonparticipating Physicians
1987	30 days	30 days
1988	19 days	26 days
1989	18 days	25 days
1990	17 days	24 days
1991	17 days	24 days
1992	17 days	24 days
1993	17 days	24 days
	Electronic Claims	Paper Claims
1994	13 days	30 days
1995	13 days	30 days

According to the regulation, interest is to be paid on claims that are not processed *and* paid within these time frames. For claims submitted after October 1, 1993, interest begins accruing as of the 31st day for electronic and paper claims. The interest rate fluctuates based on prevailing interest rates, and is generally not much more than the prime rate.

Prompt payment standards apply to clean claims only and then only to 95 percent of clean claims submitted. A clean claim is defined as a claim that does not require development; if for any reason the carrier must obtain additional information before processing the claim, it is not considered "clean."

If your claim is not paid within this time frame, contact your physician or the carrier. If the claim was assigned, your physician can contact the carrier to ask about the status of the claim. If the claim is unassigned, you will need to call the carrier to ask about the status.

Don't attempt to submit a duplicate claim; this will only cause problems. Contact the carrier or your physician to find out when the claim will be paid.

Understanding What Medicare Paid

When the Medicare carrier has made a determination on a claim, the beneficiary receives an Explanation of Medicare Benefits (EOMB) which explains the determination. The EOMB provides the beneficiary with information regarding: what services were paid for, what amount, and how much the beneficiary is expected to pay the physician or supplier.

EOMBs are sent whether the claim was assigned or unassigned, with a check included made payable to the beneficiary if the claim was unassigned. To better understand how to read your Explanation of Medicare Benefits, consider the sample shown in Figure 4-9 where the provider accepted assignment. For purposes of discussion, the form has been divided into five different areas (designated by the large numerals in Figure 4-9). Each area will be discussed separately in the following pages.

Figure 4-9: Sample Explanation of Medicare Benefits for Part B Services — *Assigned* (front page)

353204060

THIS IS NOT A BILL

Explanation of Your Medicare **Part B** Benefits

E   SMITH
450 W EAST AVE
CHICO CA 95926-7238

Summary of this notice dated	February 10, 1994	
Total charges:	$	179.00
Total Medicare approved:	$	169.00
We paid your provider:	$	55.20
Your total responsibility:	$	123.80

(1)

Your Medicare number is: 699-77-0004B   Your provider <u>accepted</u> assignment.

Details about this notice (See the back for more information.)

BILL SUBMITTED BY: Richard Anderson M.D. [F80000000]
Mailing address: Msp Test #00542, P O Box 7516,

Dates	Services and Service Codes	Charge	Medicare Approved	See Notes Below
	Claim control number 06-94040-010-010			b
Jun 24, 1993	1 other medical services [A9.?0]	$ 10.00	$ 0.00	a
Jun 24, 1993	1 Initial inpatient consult [99?.55]	+ 169.00	+ 169.00	
	Total	$ 179.00	$ 169.00	

(2)

Notes:

a   Medicare does not pay for this item or service.

b $ 100.00 was applied toward your deductible.

General Information About Medicare:

Please note that Medicare now covers flu shots.

(3)

IMPORTANT: If you have questions about this notice, call Medicare at 1-800-952-8627, or visit us at 450 West East Avenue, Chico, CA 95926. You'll need this notice when you write or call us. OUR LOMA LINDA OFFICE WILL CLOSE PERMANENTLY EFFECTIVE FEBRUARY 28, 1994.

To appeal our decision, you must WRITE to us before   August 10, 1994. See #2 on the back.

(4)

Figure 4-9 *(continued)*: Sample Explanation of Medicare Benefits
for Part B Services — *Assigned* (back page)

353204060

Page 2 of 2

E   Smith

Your Medicare number is: 699-77-0004B

More details about this notice

Here's an explanation of this notice:

Of the total charges, Medicare approved	$	169.00	Your provider agreed to accept this amount. See #4 on the back.
Less the deductible applied	-	100.00	**You have met $100.00 of your $100. deductible** for 1993.
Approved amount less deductible	$	69.00	Medicare pays 80% of this total.
Your 20%	-	13.80	You pay 20% of the approved amount
Amount after deductible and your 20%	$	55.20	
Medicare owes	$	55.20	
We are paying the provider	$	55.20	
Of the approved amount	$	169.00	
Less what Medicare owes	-	55.20	
Net responsibility	$	113.80	
Plus charges Medicare does not cover	+	10.00	You are responsible for these denied charges.
Your total responsibility	$	123.80	Your provider may bill you for this amount. If you have other insurance, the other insurance may pay this amount.

IMPORTANT: If you have questions about this notice, call Medicare at 1-800-952 -8627, or visit us at 450
West East Avenue, Chico, CA 95926. You'll need this notice when you write or call us. OUR LOMA LINDA OFFICE
WILL CLOSE PERMANENTLY EFFECTIVE FEBRUARY 28, 1994.

To appeal our decision, you must WRITE to us before   August 10, 1994. See #2 on the back.

Area 1

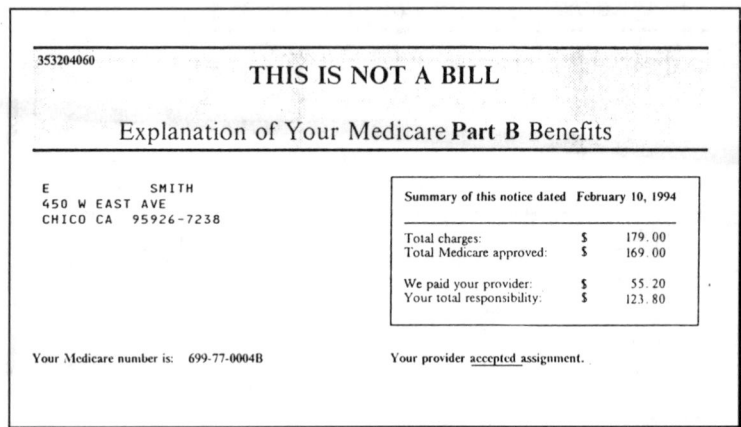

This area contains the following:

- *Disclaimer* ("This is not a bill") and *title* of notice ("Explanation of Medicare Benefits").

- *Beneficiary's name and mailing address.*

- *Beneficiary's Medicare number.*

- *Assignment status* of the claim.

- *Summary block* which summarizes information from areas 2 and 5. It includes:

  — Charges billed by the provider (total of charges for line items from Area 2).

  — Medicare's approved amount or the allowable (total of Medicare approved amounts for the line items from Area 2).

— Medicare's payment (dollar amount computed in Area 5).

— The beneficiary's payment responsibility (dollar amount computed in Area 5 appearing adjacent to "The total you are responsible for" statement).

Area 2

Details about this notice (See the back for more information.)

BILL SUBMITTED BY: Richard Anderson M.D. [F-80000000]
Mailing address: Msp Test #00542, P O Box 7516, Baltimore, MD 21207-7516

Dates	Services and Service Codes	Charge	Medicare Approved	See Notes Below
	Claim control number 06-94040-010-010			b
Jun 24, 1993	1 other medical services [A9270]	$ 10.00	$ 0.00	a
Jun 24, 1993	1 Initial inpatient consult [99255]	+ 169.00	+ 169.00	b
	Total	$ 179.00	$ 169.00	

This area contains the following:

- *Control number(s)*. These are the numbers assigned by the carrier to the claim.

- *Provider name(s) and address(es)*. This lists the physician or other provider who furnished the services. If more than one provider furnished services, they will be listed separately with the services performed by each.

- *Service or line item detail* (short descriptions and CPT and HCPCS codes). These provide the short narrative description and CPT and HCPCS codes reported by the provider. Included are the date(s) of the service(s) provided, the charge made by the physician for each service, and the amount Medicare approved (the allowable) for each service.

- *Alphabetic note codes.* The letters at the end of each line item are like footnotes providing additional information about that line item. Refer to Area 3 for the explanation associated with each letter. When the provider did not accept assignment, a statement to that affect appears at the bottom of this area.

Area 3

Notes:

a   Medicare does not pay for this item or service.

b $ 100.00 was applied toward your deductible.

General Information About Medicare:

Please note that Medicare now covers flu shots.

This area contains an alphabetic code, notes about the claim and notes about the line items in Area 2. The language in this section is uniform from carrier to carrier, provided in Section 7012 of the *Medicare Carrier's Manual*.

Area 4

IMPORTANT: If you have questions about this notice, call Medicare at 1-800-952 -8627, or visit us at 450 West East Avenue, Chico, CA 95926. You'll need this notice when you write or call us. OUR LOMA LINDA OFFICE WILL CLOSE PERMANENTLY EFFECTIVE FEBRUARY 28, 1994.

To appeal our decision, you must WRITE to us before   August 10, 1994. See #2 on the back.

Area 4 provides the carrier's name, walk-in address, and telephone number, should you wish to contact it regarding any services listed on the notice. The date by which you must request a review of any services listed on the claim is also listed in this area. See Chapter Six for information about appealing a decision on a claim.

Area 5

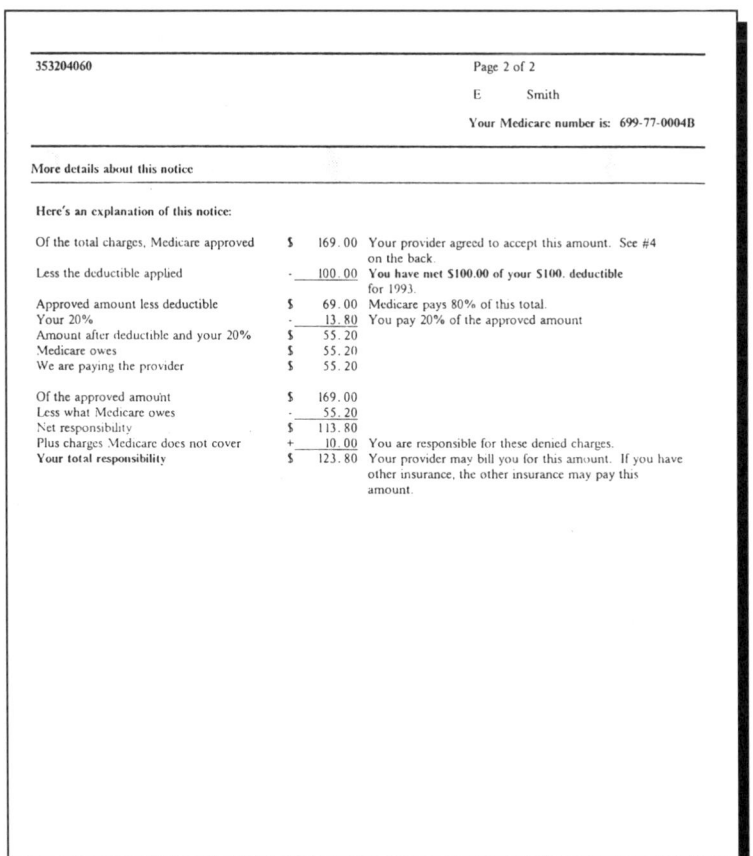

This section is "the nuts and bolts" of the statement, and probably causes the most confusion for beneficiaries. This area offers a more detailed explanation about the determination of the Medicare services than that shown in the Summary Box. The dollar amounts displayed in the Summary Box in Area 1 are derived from the computations shown in this area.

Area 5 is slightly different for assigned and unassigned claims, claims with special circumstances, or claims processed under certain circumstances (such as MSP and outpatient psychiatric treatment limitation). Also, very often all the necessary information does not fit on one page, so this area appears on page 2 of the EOMB.

- Listed first are the total charges approved, taken from the "Medicare approved" column.

- The next line is for the amount of the annual deductible applied. In Mr. Smith's case, he owes $100 to Dr. Anderson for the unpaid deductible. If Mr. Smith had satisfied $50 of the deductible from charges submitted prior to this claim, the figure in this box would be $50 and the statement would be the same.

  Note that when it says that you have met your annual deductible, this does not mean you have satisfied your obligation and therefore do not owe this amount to anyone. When the deductible amount has been fully satisfied, which means claims with approved amounts in excess of $100 have been submitted, the statement next to this line will read "You have already met the deductible for 1996." However, until this occurs, you will owe your doctor, or combination of providers, $100.

- "Approved amount less deductible" is the total approved amount less any unmet portion of the deductible. Medicare will pay 80 percent of this amount.

- "Less Medicare copayment amount" is the coinsurance amount you owe. It is 20 percent of the "approved amount less deductible" amount.

- "Amount after deductible and your 20%" is simply the difference between the coinsurance amount and the total allowed charges (less the deductible owed).

- "Medicare owes" is the amount Medicare is responsible for paying, which is 80 percent of the "approved amount less deductible." This is also the amount the carrier will pay the provider (for assigned services).

- The remaining three lines calculate again what the top lines calculated. The amount Medicare approved for payment, less what Medicare owes and will pay the provider, brings us to the "bottom line"—the amount you owe. If you have Medigap insurance, this amount may be paid by that insurer. See Chapter Five for more information about supplemental policies. Also, if the charge exceeds the limiting charge for unassigned services, this will be indicated and the correct amount will be listed. In addition, any charges for noncovered services will be added to this number to arrive at your total responsibility.

Check Summary

This page will accompany any check sent to a beneficiary for unassigned claims. If one check is sent for several claims, the payment amounts and claim control numbers will be listed on the check summary sheet. The summary will include the disclaimer, title, beneficiary name and mailing address, and beneficiary Medicare number. It also has a summary block which contains the control number; the dollar amount per control number; the total check amount; and the check number.

Note that this money is owed to your physician or other provider. You may deposit the check and then write a check to your doctor, or cash it and give the cash to your doctor. No matter how you choose to do it, remember that the money should be given to the physician.

EXAMPLES OF PART B PAYMENT

These scenarios should help you to understand how Medicare payment is calculated, and how to determine how much you must pay the physician or supplier.

1. Mrs. Jefferson visits her internist for a periodic evaluation of her diabetes and hypertension. Dr. Washington bills $60 for a Level III office visit. He is participating and so accepts assignment for the service. Medicare's allowable for this service is $40.

   a. Mrs. Jefferson has met her deductible.

   Dr. Washington's charge: $60.00
   Medicare allowable: 40.00
   Medicare pays 80% of the
     allowable to Dr. Washington: . . . . . — 32.00
   Mrs. Jefferson owes Dr. Washington
     remaining 20% coinsurance . . . . $ 8.00

b. Mrs. Jefferson has met $0 of her deductible.

Dr. Washington's charge: $60.00
Medicare allowable: 40.00
Less unpaid portion of the deductible: — 40.00
_____

Remainder: 0.00
Medicare pays 80% of the
   remaining amount to Dr. Washington: . . . 0.00
Mrs. Jefferson owes Dr.
   Washington deductible amount: $40.00

c. Mrs. Jefferson has met $85 of her deductible.

Dr. Washington's charge: $60.00
Medicare allowable: 40.00
Less unpaid portion of the deductible: — 15.00
_____

Remainder: 25.00
Medicare pays Dr. Washington
   80% of the remainder: 20.00
Mrs. Jefferson owes Dr. Washington
   remaining 20% coinsurance and
   unpaid deductible amount: $20.00

2. Mrs. Jefferson visits her family doctor because she has a sore throat. Dr. Lincoln is nonparticipating but accepts assignment for the Level II office visit. Medicare's allowable for this service is $22.89. Mrs. Jefferson has met her deductible.

Recall that Medicare will allow only 95 percent of the fee schedule amount for assigned services submitted by nonparticipating physicians. This means the allowable for this service is $21.74. Mrs. Jefferson will be required to pay only the coinsurance amount of $4.35. Medicare will send a check to Dr. Lincoln for 80 percent of the nonparticipating allowable, or $17.39.

3. Following number two above, Dr. Lincoln does not accept assignment. Medicare's allowable for the service is $22.89. The nonparticipating allowable for this service is $21.74 (95 percent of the allowable). The limiting charge is $25 (115 percent of the nonparticipating allowable).

A. Mrs. Jefferson has met her deductible.

Allowable: . . . . $ 21.74
Medicare pays Mrs. Jefferson
  80% of allowable (21.74 x .80): 17.39
Mrs. Jefferson owes Dr. Lincoln
  20% coinsurance ($4.35), the
  difference up to limiting charge
  amount ($3.26), plus the Medicare
  payment amount ($17.39): . . . . $ 25.00

B. Mrs. Jefferson has met $0 of her deductible.

Allowable: . . . . $ 21.74
Less unpaid portion of the deductible: . — 21.74

Remainder: 0.00
Medicare pays Mrs. Jefferson
  80% of remainder: 0.00
Mrs. Jefferson owes Dr. Lincoln
  the deductible plus the difference
  up to limiting charge amount: . . . . $ 25.00

C. Mrs. Jefferson has met $85 of her deductible.

Allowable: . . . . $ 21.74
Less unpaid portion of the deductible: . — 15.00

Remainder: 6.74
Medicare pays Mrs. Jefferson
80% of remainder (6.74 x .80): 5.39
Mrs. Jefferson owes Dr. Lincoln
coinsurance, deductible, and
difference up to limiting charge amount: $ 21.74

4. Mrs. Jefferson visits her internist for a periodic evaluation of her diabetes and hypertension. Dr. Washington bills $60 for a Level III office visit and $20 for her blood glucose test. He is participating and so accepts assignment for the service. Medicare's allowable for the visit is $40 and $6 for the lab test.

A week later Mrs. Jefferson visits Dr. Hancock who removes a wart from her hand. He is participating and charges $65. Medicare's allowable is $35.

A. Mrs. Jefferson has met $0 of her deductible.

- Dr. Washington's charges: . . . . $ 80.00
  Medicare allowable: 46.00
  Less amount payable at 100% (lab test): — 6.00

  Amount subject to deductible
  and coinsurance: 40.00
  Less unpaid portion of the deductible: . — 40.00

  Remainder: 0.00
  Plus amount payable at 100% (lab test): . . . 6.00

Medicare pays 80% of the remainder
plus amount payable at 100% to
Dr. Washington ($0.00 + $6.00): 6.00
Mrs. Jefferson owes Dr. Washington
deductible amount: . . . . $ 40.00

• Dr. Hancock's charge: . . . . $ 65.00
Medicare allowable: 35.00
Less unpaid portion of the deductible: . — 35.00

Remainder: 0.00
Medicare pays 80% of the remaining
amount to Dr. Hancock: 0.00
Mrs. Jefferson owes Dr. Hancock
deductible amount: $35.00

Mrs. Jefferson still owes $25.00 ($100 - $40 - $35) of her deductible that must be paid before Medicare will begin paying benefits. Once this amount is satisfied through submission of another charge and she pays this amount to the appropriate party, then Medicare will begin paying 80 percent of the charges approved for payment.

B. Mrs. Jefferson has met $50 of her deductible.

• Dr. Washington's charge: . . . . $ 60.00
Medicare allowable: 40.00

Amount subject to deductible
and coinsurance: 40.00
Less unpaid portion of the deductible: . — 40.00

Remainder: 0.00

Plus amount payable at 100% (lab test): . . + 6.00
Medicare pays 80% of the remaining
   amount plus amount payable at 100%
   to Dr. Washington (.80 X $0) + $6: . . . . $ 6.00

Mrs. Jefferson owes Dr. Washington
   deductible amount: . . . . $ 40.00

- Dr. Hancock's charge: . . . . $ 65.00
Medicare allowable: 35.00
Less unpaid portion of the deductible: . — 10.00

Remainder: 25.00
Medicare pays 80% of the remaining
   amount to Dr. Hancock: 20.00
Mrs. Jefferson owes Dr. Hancock deductible
   amount ($10) and coinsurance ($5): . . . $15.00

5. Mr. Adams is admitted to the hospital for a triple coronary artery bypass. His cardiovascular surgeon, Dr. Madison, participates with Medicare and so accepts assignment for the surgery.

   Dr. Madison's charge is $9,000. Medicare's allowable is $3,200. Dr. Truman, also a participating physician, assists with the surgery. His charge is $1,800. Dr. Eisenhower administers the anesthesia for which he charges $1,200. Medicare's allowable is $600. Mr. Adams has met his Part B deductible.

• Dr. Madison's charge: . . . . $ 9,000.00
Medicare allowable: 3,200.00
Medicare pays 80% of allowable
  to Dr. Madison: . . . . — 2,560.00

Mr. Adams owes Dr. Madison coinsurance: $ 640.00

• Dr. Truman's charge: . . . . $ 1,800.00
Medicare allowable (16% of allowable): . . 512.00
Medicare pays 80% of allowable
  to Dr. Truman: 409.60

Mr. Adams owes Dr. Truman coinsurance: $ 102.40

• Dr. Eisenhower's charge: . . . . $ 1,200.00
Medicare allowable: 600.00
Medicare pays 80% of allowable
  to Dr. Eisenhower: 480.00
Mr. Adams owes
  Dr. Eisenhower coinsurance: . . . . $ 120.00

• Total out-of-pocket costs: ($640.00
  to Dr. Madison + 102.40 to Dr. Truman
  + 120.00 to Dr. Eisenhower) . . . . $ 862.40

Payment includes all services related to the follow-up treatment by Dr. Madison, including visits in and out of the hospital, for 90 days following surgery.

Note that for Part A, Mr. Adams will also be required to pay the inpatient hospital deductible of $736 to the hospital for his stay (assuming he has not exceeded 60 days in a benefit period).

6. Mr. Coolidge entered an ambulatory surgical center (ASC) for drainage of his kidney required because of a renal vascular disorder. His physician, Dr. Taylor, participated with Medicare and charged $2,200 for the procedure. Medicare's allowable is $780. Mr. Coolidge has met his deductible.

The ASC will charge Mr. Coolidge for use of the facility. The ASC facility charge is based upon the procedure performed. Procedures approved for performance in an ASC are classified into eight payment groups, each with a set allowable (similar in idea to the way hospitals are paid). For this example, this procedure is classified into the ASC payment group for which the allowable is $515.

Dr. Taylor's charge: . . . . $ 2,200.00
Medicare allowable: 780.00
Medicare pays 80% of allowable
   to Dr. Taylor: 624.00
Mr. Coolidge owes Dr. Taylor
   coinsurance: . . . . $ 156.00

ASC facility rate: . . . . $ 515.00
Medicare allowable: 515.00
Medicare pays 80% of allowable to the ASC: 412.00
Mr. Coolidge owes the ASC coinsurance: $ 103.00

7. Mrs. Roosevelt went to see Dr. Nixon complaining of a sore throat and headache. Dr. Nixon, wanting to be thorough, discussed Mrs. Roosevelt's complete medical and family history, and examined not only her throat, but also listened to her lungs and heart, took blood pressure, and briefly examined other body systems. He discussed treatment options (bed rest, fluids, aspirin).

For this extensive exam, Dr. Nixon billed a Level V (the highest level) office visit. When Mrs. Roosevelt received her bill, she noticed that the Medicare carrier had changed the code for her service, thereby "down-coding" the service to a Level II visit. The reason for this is that the carrier did not feel that the diagnosis ofsore throat justified such an extensive level of service, but it would justify a more basic level.

Therefore, Mrs. Roosevelt is responsible for the coinsurance (and unmet deductible) due for the lesser level of service. Dr. Nixon must accept the Medicare allowable for the lesser level of service as payment in full (he accepted assignment); he may not collect the difference from Mrs. Ford or her supplemental insurer.

Had Dr. Nixon been nonparticipating, the same rule would still apply: he may collect only up to the Medicare limiting charge for the lesser level of service.

8. Mrs. Truman visited Dr. Taylor, her family doctor, for her annual physical examination. Dr. Taylor is participating with Medicare and so accepts assignment.

   Included in the exam is a screening pap smear. In addition, Mrs. Truman asks to receive a Vitamin B_{12} shot. Her friends have told her it would make her feel better. Dr. Taylor agrees to administer the B_{12} since it cannot do her any harm. But he informs her that Medicare does not consider Vitamin B_{12} shots to be a reasonable and necessary treatment and so will not pay for it. He asks her to sign a notice that explains this and includes an agreement that she will pay for the injection if Medicare denies payment.

   He charges $125 for the visit, $10 for the pap smear, and $70 for the Vitamin B_{12} shot. Mrs. Truman has met $75 of her deductible.

Medicare does not pay for the annual physical exam because routine care is not covered. However, Medicare will allow payment for the screening pap smear because Mrs. Truman has met the qualifications for payment of this screening test. Medicare's allowable for the pap smear is $7.

Mrs. Truman's EOMB also indicates that the Vitamin B_{12} shot was indeed not covered, and that, since the doctor provided advance notice that Medicare might not pay, she is responsible for payment of the injection. Since this service is not covered, Dr. Taylor can charge his usual fee for the injection.

Dr. Taylor's charges:	$ 205.00
Medicare allowable:	7.00
Less amount payable at 100% (lab test):	— 7.00
Amount subject to deductible and coinsurance:	0.00
Amount payable at 100% (lab test):	7.00
Medicare pays 100% of lab test to Dr. Taylor:	7.00
Mrs. Truman owes Dr. Taylor for noncovered service ($125) plus Vitamin B_{12} shot ($70):	$ 195.00

In addition to her Medicare coverage, Mrs. Truman has a supplemental policy that pays for preventive care. The denial from Medicare is submitted directly from the Medicare carrier to the supplemental policy insurer (because Dr. Taylor accepted assignment).

The maximum benefit for preventive care is $120, payment of which is based on the Medicare allowable amount. Since the Medicare allowable for the service (were it a visit for a medical condition rather than just a "check-up") is $80, her supplemental insurer will pay Dr. Taylor $80. He cannot attempt to collect more than this amount from Mrs. Truman. He is still bound by the terms of assignment in which he agrees to accept Medicare's allowable charge as payment in full. (See Chapter Five for more information about insurance to supplement Medicare coverage.) Mrs. Truman also owes Dr. Taylor $70 for the vitamin injection.

9. Mr. Grant was treated by his physician, Dr. Lincoln, because he burned his hand at work. Dr. Lincoln charges $90 for the treatment and accepts assignment on the claim. The bill was submitted to the Workers' Compensation carrier, which approved $85 for the treatment and paid 80 percent of that amount, or $68. Since Medicare is the secondary payer, the bill is then submitted to Medicare. Medicare's allowable for this service is $40.

To calculate secondary payments, Medicare uses a four-step process:

1. Calculate the amount billed minus the amount paid by the primary insurer ($90 — $68 = $22).

2. Calculate the amount Medicare would pay if it was the primary insurer ($40 x .80 = $32).

3. Compare the primary insurer's and Medicare's allowables. Choose the higher amount. Then determine the difference between the amount chosen and the amount paid by the primary insurer ($85 — $68 = $17)

4. Medicare will pay the lowest of the amounts calculated in steps 1, 2, and 3 (= $17).

Medicare will pay Dr. Lincoln $17, which is the full amount of the copayment as determined by the Workers' Compensation carrier's allowable for the service. Mr. Grant, then, will pay nothing from his own funds. (For more information about Medicare as Secondary Payer, refer to Chapter Nine.)

CHAPTER 5

MEDIGAP POLICIES, PRIVATE HEALTH PLANS, AND MANAGED CARE PLANS

Medicare provides basic protection against many costs of health care, but does not pay all medical expenses. It also does not cover most long-term care expenses. Because of these "gaps" in coverage, many private insurance companies sell insurance to supplement Medicare, called Medigap insurance, as well as separate long-term care insurance.

Instead of the standard fee-for-service Medicare and Medigap policies, beneficiaries may elect to enroll in a managed care plan, such as an HMO. Managed care plans contract with the Health Care Financing Administration (HCFA) to provide a set of services to Medicare-eligible persons. Medicare will pay the plan a preset premium for each Medicare beneficiary enrolled in the plan. The plan then provides all care to the persons enrolled in the plan.

As you may be learning, there are many Medigap and managed care plans available to seniors. Making the decision about what type of plan is best for you includes considering factors other than just cost. It is for this reason this chapter reviews the Medigap plans available, discusses the actual benefits provided, and helps you walk through the process of choosing the best plan for you. Also included in this chapter is a discussion of managed care options and what those options can mean for you.

THE GAPS IN MEDICARE COVERAGE

Before moving to a discussion of the types of additional insurance coverage available to supplement Medicare coverage, it is important to remember what Medicare does not pay for—that is, what you are responsible for paying. This includes deductibles and coinsurance as well as noncovered services. The beneficiary's financial responsibility under each type of coverage is outlined below.

Inpatient Hospital Care

You pay:

- Inpatient hospital deductible of $736 per benefit period.

- Coinsurance of $184 per day for days 61-90 of a hospital stay (totaling $5,520).

- All charges for coverage after day 90 unless you use lifetime reserve days.

- Coinsurance of $368 per day for each lifetime reserve day used (totaling $22,080).

- First three pints of whole blood or packed cells used in each year.

- Private hospital room and private nurse (unless medically necessary).

- Personal convenience items, such as a telephone or television in your room.

- Non-emergency care in a nonparticipating hospital.

- Care received outside the United States.

Psychiatric Hospital Care

You pay:

- Same as for inpatient hospital care.

- All charges for care after 190 days of this type of care in your lifetime.

Skilled Nursing Facility Care

You pay:

- Coinsurance of $92 per day for days 21 through 100 in each benefit period (totaling $7,360).

- All charges for care after day 100 in each benefit period.

- All charges for care that is less than the level of care Medicare covers in a SNF.

- All costs if you were not transferred to the SNF in a timely manner after a qualifying hospital stay.

- All charges for care in a general nursing home, or in a SNF not approved by Medicare, or custodial care provided by a Medicare-approved SNF.

- Blood deductible.

Home Health Care

You pay:

- All charges for full-time nursing care.

- All charges for meals delivered to your home.

- All charges for drugs.

- Coinsurance of 20 percent of approved charges for durable medical equipment.

- Charges for homemaker services that are primarily to assist you in meeting personal care or housekeeping needs.

Hospice Care

You pay:

- Prescription drugs for pain relief and symptom management, for which you can be charges five percent of the reasonable cost, but no more than $5 per prescription.

- Respite care, for which you can be charged about $5 per day.

- Deductibles and coinsurance when regular Medicare benefits are used for treatment of a condition other than the terminal illness.

Physician and Supplier Care

You pay:

- Annual deductible of $100.

- Coinsurance of 20 percent for Medicare-approved charges, and balance billing amount (up to limiting charge amount).

- 50 percent of Medicare-approved amounts for most outpatient mental health treatment.

- All charges for:

  — independent physical or occupational therapists' services in excess of Medicare's $900 annual maximum

  — services determined to be not reasonable and necessary

  — most self-administrable prescription drugs and immunizations, except for pneumococcal, influenza, and hepatitis B vaccinations

— routine physicals and other screening services, except for mammograms and pap smears

— routine eye examinations or eyeglasses (except prosthetic lenses after cataract surgery).

— acupuncture treatment

— most chiropractic care

— most dental care and dentures

— hearing aids or routine hearing loss examinations

— care provided outside the United States

— routine foot care except when a medical condition affecting the lower limbs (such as diabetes) requires care by a medical professional

— services of naturopaths, Christian Science practitioners, immediate relatives, or members of your household

• First three pints of blood.

As you saw in the examples provided in Chapters Two and Three, the amounts you may have to pay out of your own pocket can accumulate rapidly. So unless you are independently wealthy or like taking chances, it is likely that you will need additional insurance to help pay for expenses, services, and supplies that Medicare covers only partially or does not cover at all.

MEDIGAP POLICIES

Insurance policies which fill the "gaps" in Medicare coverage are called Medigap policies. Both state and federal laws govern sales of Medigap insurance. Policies designed for this purpose must be specifically identified as Medicare supplemental policies. Other kinds of insurance are available that may help you with out-of-pocket health care expenses, such as nursing home or long-term care insurance or specified disease policies (e.g., cancer insurance that pays for services related only to treatment of specific kinds of cancer), but these plans do not qualify as Medigap plans.

Companies or agents selling Medigap insurance must avoid certain illegal practices. Federal criminal and civil penalties may be imposed against any insurance company or agent that knowingly:

• Sells a policy that duplicates Medicare coverage, Medicaid coverage, or private health insurance coverage.

• Uses high pressure tactics to force or frighten a beneficiary into buying a Medigap policy or to make fraudulent or misleading comparisons to induce the beneficiary to switch from one company or policy to another.

• Says that they are employees or agents of the Medicare program or of any government agency.

- Makes a false statement that a policy meets legal standards for certification when it does not.

- Denies the beneficiary his Medigap open enrollment period by refusing to issue a policy, placing conditions on the policy, or discriminating in the price of the policy because of the beneficiary's health status, claims experience, receipt of health care, or medical condition.

- Uses the U.S. mail for advertising or delivering Medigap policies in a state if the policies have not been approved for sale in that state.

It is also illegal for anyone to sell you a Medigap plan that does not conform to the standardization requirements. This includes any special arrangements with a physician, such as a "retainer agreement," where he agrees to provide certain non-Medicare-covered services and waive the Medicare coinsurance and deductible amounts. If a doctor refuses to see you as a Medicare patient unless you pay him an annual fee and/or sign one of these retainer agreements, file a complaint with federal authorities by calling 1-800-638-6833.

Standardization

During 1992, to make it easier for consumers to comparison shop, most states adopted regulations limiting the sale of Medigap insurance to no more than ten standard plans. The plans were developed by the National Association of Insurance Commissioners and were incorporated into state and federal law.

For ease of reference, each plan is designated with a letter, A through J; policy A is the basic policy offering a "core package" of benefits and J is the most comprehensive package, offering benefits which pay for services not covered or not fully covered by Medicare. The other nine policies each have a different combination of benefits, but all include the core package.

The basic policy is available in all states. Insurance companies are prohibited from changing the combination of benefits available or from changing the letter designation of any of the plans.

Each state is required to sell Plan A and all Medigap insurers must make Plan A available if they are going to sell any Medigap plans in a state. While not required to make any of the other nine plans available, most insurers offer several plans to pick from, and some offer all ten. The insurer can independently decide which plan(s) it will sell as long as the plan(s) chosen are approved for sale in the state in which it is to be sold. Some states do not allow the sale of all ten plans, such as Delaware which does not allow the sale of Plans C, F, G, and H and Vermont which prohibits the sale of Plans F, G, and I.

Medigap insurers must use the same format, language, and definitions in describing the benefits of each Medigap plan. They are also required to use a uniform chart and outline of coverage to summarize the benefits. This chart is shown in Figure 5-1. The discussion of each of the benefits under each plan follows the chart.

States are also permitted to allow an insurer to add "new and innovative" benefits to a plan that otherwise complies with applicable standards. These benefits must be cost-effective, not otherwise available in the marketplace, and offered in a manner that is consistent with the goal of simplification. Contact your state insurance department to find out whether any new and innovative benefits are available in your state.

Minnesota, Massachusetts, and Wisconsin had alternative Medigap standardization programs in effect before passage of the federal law and so may have slightly different plans from those sold in other states. If you live in one of these states, contact your state insurance department to find out what coverage is available.

Enrollment

The open enrollment period for selecting Medigap policies guarantees that for a period of up to six months from the date you are both enrolled in Medicare Part B and age 65, you cannot be denied Medigap insurance or charged higher premiums because of health problems. You have the right to buy a Medigap policy of your choice regardless of any health problems you have. Note, however, that even though beneficiaries are guaranteed enrollment, the Medigap policy may not provide services for preexisting conditions until a six-month waiting period has passed. Even if the person buys a Medigap policy and switches to another within the six-month period, the open enrollment guarantee is still in effect.

The open enrollment period also applies to those persons who work and retain health insurance coverage through their (or their spouse's) employer. Once the employer policy terminates, the beneficiary may apply for Medigap insurance. Enrollment is guaranteed for six months from the date of *enrollment* in Part B, not eligibility for Part B. The insurer can exclude preexisting conditions from coverage for a period of up to six months.

Effective January 1, 1995, beneficiaries enrolled in Medicare on the basis of disability also have a six-month open enrollment period when they turn 65.

Premiums

Although benefits for each Medigap plan are standard, premiums are not. Premiums are set by the insurer selling the plan, under approval by the state in which the plans are sold. The insurer can use three methods of setting premiums:

1. If the insurer uses the *issue age method* and you were age 65 when you bought the policy, you will always pay the same premium the company charges people age 65, regardless of your age.

2. If the insurer uses the *attained age method*, the premium is based on your current age and will increase as you grow older.

3. If the insurer uses the *no age rating method*, everyone pays the same premium regardless of age.

The insurer can raise premiums only when it has approval from the state insurance department to do so for everyone else with the same policy.

Premiums can range from as little as $30 per month for the basic Plan A package to as much as $150 per month for the comprehensive Plan J package. Before deciding which package best suits your needs, you will need to decide if the premium paid is worth the amount of the benefit.

Renewal and Review Period

All standard Medigap policies are guaranteed renewable. This means that the insurer cannot refuse to renew your policy unless you fail to pay the premiums or you made a material misrepresentation (lied) on the policy. Note, however, that policies sold prior to the standardization may allow the company to refuse to renew the policy on an individual basis.

Medigap policies also carry a "30-day money back guarantee" called the free-look provision. This means the insurer must give you at least 30 days to review a Medigap policy. If you decide you don't want it, return it to the company (or agent) within 30 days of receiving it and request a refund for all premiums paid.

If you have a Medigap policy for at least six months and decide to switch to a different policy, the replacement policy cannot impose a waiting period for a preexisting condition *unless* a benefit is included in the new policy that was not included in the old policy. The insurer can impose a waiting period of up to six months for that particular benefit.

Medigap insurers also are not required to issue a policy after the six-month open enrollment period expires. However, since these policies are the insurer's line of business, it is likely that the insurer would still issue a policy, albeit with a clause to exclude certain pre-existing conditions.

Medigap Policies Sold Before Standardization

Many of the federal requirements governing Medigap plans do not apply to policies sold before the standardization in 1992. You are generally not required to switch to a standard plan unless the older plan does not have a renewal guarantee and the company discontinues the plan you have. However, even though you're not required to switch, you may want to consider doing so, if it is to your advantage financially and another insurer is willing to sell you a policy. This will guarantee your benefits and the renewability of the policy.

If you do switch, you will not be allowed to go back to the old policy. Be sure to evaluate the benefit of switching before doing so, including comparing benefits and premiums, and determining if there are any waiting periods before coverage will begin. Some of the older policies provided better coverage of prescription drugs and extended SNF care.

Also, you will be required to sign a statement that you are replacing an existing policy and that you will not keep both policies. You do not need more than one policy. Do not, however, cancel the existing policy until the new one is in force and you have decided to keep it. Canceling prematurely may cause you to lose benefits or undergo a waiting period for previously uninsured benefits.

Summary of Ten Standard Medigap Plans

Figure 5-1 outlines the benefits provided under the ten standard Medigap plans. As shown in the table, these plans offer a combination of up to nine benefits (12 benefits if you divide the "Basic Benefit" into its four parts). Each of the benefits is described below.

Plan A provides the core package, or "Basic Benefit," which includes the first four benefits described below. Plan J includes all 12 benefits. Every company must make Plan A available. Some plans may not be available in specific states.

Figure 5-1: The 10 Standard Medicare Supplement Plans

A	B	C	D	E
Basic Benefit	Basic Benefit	Basic Benefit	Basic Benefit	Basic Benefit
		Skilled Nursing Coinsurance	Skilled Nursing Coinsurance	Skilled Nursing Coinsurance
	Part A Deductible	Part A Deductible	Part A Deductible	Part A Deductible
		Part B Deductible		
		Foreign Travel Emergency	Foreign Travel Emergency	Foreign Travel Emergency
			At-Home Recovery	
				Preventive Care

1. *Basic Benefit: Part A inpatient hospital coinsurance*—pays the hospital coinsurance, at $184 per day, for days 61 through 90 of a hospital stay in a single benefit period and, for stays over 90 days, coinsurance at $368 per day, for lifetime reserve days used in a benefit period.

Figure 5-1 *(cont.)*: The 10 Standard Medicare Supplement Plans

F	G	H	I	J
Basic Benefit	Basic Benefit	Basic Benefit	Basic Benefit	Basic Benefit
Skilled Nursing Coinsurance	Skilled Nursing Coinsurance	Skilled Nursing Coinsurance	Skilled Nursing Coinsurance	Skilled Nursing Coinsurance
Part A Deductible	Part A Deductible	Part A Deductible	Part A Deductible	Part A Deductible
Part B Deductible				Part B Deductible
Part B Excess (100%)	Part B Excess (100%)		Part B Excess (100%)	Part B Excess (100%)
Foreign Travel Emergency	Foreign Travel Emergency	Foreign Travel Emergency	Foreign Travel Emergency	Foreign Travel Emergency
	At-Home Recovery		At-Home Recovery	At-Home Recovery
		Basic Drug Benefit ($1250 limit)	Basic Drug Benefit ($1250 limit)	Basic Drug Benefit ($1250 limit)
				Preventive Care

2. *Basic Benefit: Additional 365 inpatient hospital days*—covers out-of-pocket costs for hospital stays longer than 150 days since Medicare will help cover costs for stays up to only 150 days. The additional 365 days are for a lifetime, which means they are not renewable after a benefit period or

each calendar year. Payment is made for Medicare-covered services at the Medicare payment rate. The beneficiary has no coinsurance responsibility in conjunction with this benefit.

3. *Basic Benefit: Part B coinsurance*—pays the 20 percent coinsurance amount (or 50 percent of approved charges for outpatient mental health services) due for physician and other medical services, including durable medical equipment. Recall that the coinsurance amount is the difference between Medicare's allowable charge and the 80 percent amount Medicare pays to the physician (for assigned services) or the beneficiary (for unassigned services).

4. *Basic Benefit: Blood deductible*—pays the annual blood deductible, which is for the first three pints of blood used and not replaced each year. The blood deductible is satisfied for both Parts A *and* B when it is met for either one.

5. *Part A inpatient hospital deductible*—pays for the inpatient hospital deductible of $736 per benefit period.

6. *Skilled Nursing Facility coinsurance*—pays for the Part A coinsurance of $92 per day for days 21 through 100 in a single benefit period for post-hospital SNF care.

7. *Part B annual deductible*—covers the Part B deductible which is $100 per year.

8. *Foreign travel emergency*— pays for 80 percent of charges for emergency care received in a foreign country during the first 60 days of a trip outside the U.S..The beneficiary is responsible for a $250 per calendar year deductible; the lifetime maximum benefit is $50,000. This benefit fills the gap created because Medicare does not cover care provided outside the United States (except certain emergency and urgent care in certain circumstances).

9. *At-home recovery*—covers those services not covered by Medicare to provide short-term, at-home assistance with activities of daily living for those recovering from an illness, injury, or surgery. The maximum benefit is $1,600 per calendar year. To qualify for this benefit, you must receive Medicare-covered home health services after an illness, injury, or surgery, and the services must be ordered by your doctor.

10. *Preventive care*—provides coverage for preventive health services not covered by Medicare, subject to a $120 maximum annual benefit. The screening services must be ordered by a physician. Note that the maximum benefit is the maximum amount the supplemental insurer will pay based on the Medicare allowable for the preventive services. In other words, if the doctor's charge is $120 but the Medicare allowable is only $80 for the service, the insurer will pay $80. The doctor is still limited to collecting up to the Medicare allowable amount (or limiting charge amount) for that service. Also, there is no coinsurance due from the beneficiary; the

supplemental insurer pays 100 percent of the allowable amount.

11. *Part B excess*—covers either 80 or 100 percent (depending on the plan) of Part B excess charges, which represent the difference between the doctor's actual charge as billed, not to exceed any charge limitation established by the Medicare program or state law (i.e., the limiting charge), and the Medicare allowable. In other words, this benefit pays for the beneficiary's out-of-pocket liability for the limiting charge and may pay the difference between the physician's actual charge and the Medicare allowable for assigned services.

12. *Prescription drugs*—pays 50 percent of outpatient prescription drug charges not covered by Medicare, subject to a $250 per calendar year deductible and a maximum $1,250 (or $3,000) in benefits per calendar year.

Weighing the Benefits

Now that you understand the benefits provided by the Medigap plans, you must determine which combination of benefits best suits your needs. While you may be tempted to go for the comprehensive coverage offered by Plan J, it may be more than you need. Let's go through each benefit, with a viewpoint of how much "benefit" it actually provides.

• The core package includes the four basic benefits: *inpatient hospital coinsurance, coverage for additional 365 days of inpatient hospital care, the*

Part B coinsurance, and the *blood deductible.* The possible out-of-pocket liability for the inpatient hospital deductible and coinsurance is $28,336, plus daily hospital charges for 365 days of care plus blood and 20 percent of physician and supplier charges. This number could be well in excess of $250,000 in the event of a catastrophic illness. Since the average price of Plan A is about $40 per month, the protection it affords is well worth the price.

• The next two benefits seem to be equally well justified. The *inpatient hospital deductible* benefit is for a minimum of $736 per year. If more than one benefit period is used in a year, the benefit would be greater. If the premium is only $8 more per month, or $96 per year, it would seem that this is a worthwhile benefit. The same is true for the benefit for *skilled nursing facility coinsurance,* which could amount to $7,360 per benefit period. An additional $5 or $10 or even $15 per month would justify purchase of this benefit.

• The benefits for payment of the *Part B deductible* and 80 percent *foreign travel emergency payment* are not quite so clear. The Part B deductible is only $100 per year. The premium increase should therefore be no more than $8 per month to justify this. If you do not travel abroad, or even to Canada or Mexico, the foreign travel emergency benefit may be unnecessary. Also, the benefit is capped at $50,000 per lifetime.

- The *at-home recovery* benefit is capped at $1,600 annually, with visits capped at $40 per day. This means the Medigap plan will pay for 40 visits, or 5 weeks and 5 days. Be sure the increase in premiums is not so much that it negates the benefit.

- The *Part B excess benefit* will limit your out-of-pocket costs. However, compare the cost of the increased premium for this benefit with the actual cost of the services you are purchasing. The premium should be lower than what you would expect to spend on these services.

Preventive Care and Prescription Drugs: Take a Careful Look

The last two benefits, *preventive care* and the *prescription drug* benefit, deserve special attention. Many beneficiaries think these two benefits look especially appealing. However, since both are capped, this may not be true. Let's consider an example.

Mr. Francisco takes blood pressure medication and medication for an ulcer; his medication expenses amount to $80 per month. Since he is in his 60s, his doctor recommends an annual sigmoidoscopy to screen for colon cancer, for which his doctor charges $250. He is considering buying either comprehensive Medigap Plan J or Plan G. To decide which makes most sense for him, Mr. Francisco begins by calculating what he spends each year on medication and on preventive care (the benefits covered by Plan J but not by Plan G).

Medication at $80 per month	$ 960
Preventive care	$ 250
Total	$1,210

He next must calculate what Plan J would pay and what he would be required to pay for these services.

Medication: 50 percent up to a maximum of $3,000 per year; $250 deductible:

$960 - $250 deductible =	$ 710
$710 x .50 payment =	balance of $ 355
add $250 (deductible)	+ $ 250
Total owed by Mr. Francisco	$ 605

Preventive care: $120 maximum

Charge	$ 250
Medicare allowable	$ 90
Payment by supplemental insurer	$ 90
Total owed by Mr. Francisco	$ 0

Mr. Francisco's total expense for prescription drugs and preventive care under Plan J would be: $605 + $0 = $605. The only additional benefit offered by Plan J that is not offered by Plan G is the Part B deductible, at $100 per year. Now Mr. Francisco can determine his savings under Plan J:

Mr. Francisco's costs:		Costs under Plan J:	
Medication	$ 960	Medication	$ 605
Preventive care	$ 250	Preventive care	$ 0
Part B deductible	$ 100	Part B deductible	$ 0
Total	$1,310	Total	$ 650

If Mr. Francisco chooses Plan J over Plan G, he would save $705 ($1,310 - $605) per year. But the policy costs him $65 more per month, or $780 per year. So, even though the plan has more benefits, Mr. Francisco finds that it really would not benefit him at all, since the premiums would cost him more than he would save. If, however, Mr. Francisco thought he might need more medication in the future, he might consider the coverage since it would save him money as he spent more on prescription drugs.

PURCHASE CONSIDERATIONS

Some factors to consider when buying a Medigap plan:

1. *Price*—The most compelling reason for choosing a company will probably be price. Companies can vary greatly in their prices for the same plan, so shop around and compare premiums. You may find a bargain. In addition, while the American Association of Retired Persons (AARP), a well-known and very large association of seniors, often provides the lowest rates, this is not always true. Compare your quote from AARP with other insurers in your state to be sure you are getting the best price.

   Realize also that while a policy using the attained age method for setting premiums may initially be less expensive than other policies, it may be that policies using other methods of setting premiums may be less expensive after a few years. Keep this is mind when comparing prices.

2. *Service*—This is probably the second most important factor after price. Try to find out about the company's reputation for service. Call the customer service line to find out how long you have to wait before speaking to a representative. Assess how helpful, friendly, and knowledgeable the representatives appear to be. Talk with other customers to learn about their experiences. You'll probably be dealing with this company for a long time, so you want to feel comfortable that they will serve you just as well after you buy your policy as before.

3. *Claims submission*—Under certain circumstances, you may not have to file a claim with your Medigap insurer. By law, the Medicare carrier that processes claims in your area must send your claim to a Medigap insurer when the following three conditions are met: (1) your physician or supplier is participating with Medicare (and accepted assignment); (2) your policy is a Medigap policy; and (3) you instructed your physician or supplier to indicate on the claim form that you wish payment of Medigap benefits to be made to the participating physician or supplier.

The physician or supplier should include your Medigap policy number on the Medicare claim form. When these conditions are met, the Medicare carrier will send the processed claim to the Medigap insurer and send you the Explanation of Medicare Benefits (EOMB). Your Medigap insurer will then process your claim and send you a notice that benefits have been paid to your physician or supplier.

Under another arrangement, Medigap insurers have "crossover" contracts with Medicare carriers whereby the carrier will send all Medigap claims to that insurer, or crossover the claims, regardless of the physician's participation status. You are not responsible for filing any claims. To find out whether your Medigap insurer has a crossover contract, contact the local Medicare carrier or ask the Medigap insurer.

4. *Payment time*—Find out the turnaround time for payment of benefits by your Medigap insurer. You know that Medicare law governs the amount of time the carrier must hold clean claims before paying them. However, no such laws govern Medigap plans. While most are reasonable (paying within 30 days), it would be wise to request this information so you are not stuck paying costs out of your pocket with no hope of reimbursement for more than 30 days.

5. *Insurer's reputation*—Insurance companies are not created equal. Before you choose one, find out about the company's reputation, especially related to service and payment time. Talk to friends about their companies. Ask the insurance company to provide information about its service and strength.

Medicare SELECT

In addition to the standard Medigap policies, a new kind of Medigap insurance was introduced in 1992 called Medicare SELECT. The difference between SELECT and standard Medigap insurance is that beneficiaries agree to use the services of certain hospitals and physicians ("preferred providers") in return for lower premiums. If the beneficiary chooses to use a provider who is not part of the SELECT panel of preferred providers for other than emergency services, the Medigap insurer may not pay anything. Medicare, however, will pay its standard share of approved expenses.

Medicare SELECT was designed as an experimental program and was initially offered in only 16 states (Alabama, Arizona, California, Florida, Illinois, Indiana, Kentucky, Massachusetts, Michigan, Minnesota, Missouri, North Dakota, Ohio, Texas, Washington, and Wisconsin). The law originating the SELECT program allowed it only through June 1995. Public Law 104-18, passed in 1995, authorized continuance of the program until the year 2005 and expanded availability to include all 50 states.

OTHER TYPES OF INSURANCE

In addition to Medigap plans, there are other types of insurance that you can consider purchasing for services not covered by Medicare and not covered by Medigap plans. These policies are not designed to bridge the gaps in Medicare coverage. Coverage is usually limited to a specific type of service or for a specific kind of illness.

While these policies can be helpful in the event of a catastrophic problem, be sure they actually pay for the care you think they pay for, such as nursing home care, and do not have a very low ceiling on the dollar amount of benefits they will pay. Research these plans carefully, be aware of what you are buying, and be sure you need this additional coverage before you buy the policy.

These policies may also duplicate some Medicare or Medigap benefits you already have. Insurers must provide you with a statement describing any duplication of benefits. These policies do not have to conform to the laws governing Medigap policies whereby the insurer cannot sell you a policy that duplicates Medicare benefits. So check these policies very carefully and be sure you are not paying for the same thing twice.

Specified disease insurance provides benefits for a single disease or group of related diseases, such as cancer. The value of the policy lies in the possibility that you will actually get the disease specified. Benefits are usually limited to payment of a fixed amount for each type of treatment. Remember, also, that Medicare and Medigap plans will very likely cover many of the costs associated with any disease you contract.

Hospital indemnity insurance pays a fixed cash amount for each day you are hospitalized up to a set number of days. Some policies may have added benefits such as surgical benefits or SNF benefits. Some policies also have a maximum number of days or a maximum payment amount covered under the policy. Again, unless you anticipate being confined to a hospital for more than 515 days (Medicare's maximum of 150 days plus additional 365 days under a Medigap plan), this coverage would probably not be needed.

Long-term care insurance is available for custodial care provided in a nursing home. Since Medicare and Medigap policies do not pay for custodial care (which is the type of care most patients in nursing homes require), this type of policy could be beneficial. Some of these policies also cover home care and others pay for SNF care, even if Medicare benefits are not available.

Before purchasing a policy of this type, be sure it does not duplicate coverage provided by Medicare and a Medigap policy or that it does not rely on other coverage to make a determination of coverage. Verify what types of nursing homes and services are covered by the plan. You can request a copy of *A Shopper's Guide to Long-Term Care Insurance* from either your state insurance department or the National Association of Insurance Commissioners, 120 West 12th Street, Suite 1100, Kansas City, MO 64105-1925. In addition, HCFA has a publication titled *Guide to Choosing a Nursing Home*, which you can obtain by writing to Medicare Publications, HCFA, 6325 Security Boulevard, Baltimore, MD 21207. Other books, including *Making the Nursing Home Decision*, can be obtained in local book stores.

MANAGED CARE

Managed care plans are sometimes called coordinated care plans, prepaid plans, or HMOs (health maintenance organizations). Think of them as a combination insurance company and doctor/hospital. Like an insurance company, they cover health care costs in return for monthly premium and, like a doctor or hospital, they provide health care services.

Each plan has its own group of health care providers, including physicians and hospitals, who generally offer comprehensive, coordinated medical services to plan members (enrollees) on a prepaid basis. Services usually must be obtained from the professionals and facilities that are part of the plan. Depending upon how the plan is organized, the services are either provided at one or more centrally located health facility or in the private practice offices of the professionals affiliated with the plan.

Managed care plans enter into a contract with HCFA to provide Medicare-covered services to enrolled Medicare beneficiaries. HCFA pays the plan a monthly premium for each Medicare beneficiary, which represents 95 percent of Medicare's share of the cost of the services received by each Medicare beneficiary. In return, the beneficiary does not pay the Medicare deductible and coinsurance for Medicare-covered services provided by the plan. Instead, the plan is permitted to charge the beneficiary a monthly premium, and/or nominal copayments when services are received.

Usually the plan makes no additional charges no matter how many times you see your physician, are hospitalized, or use other covered services. The only requirement is that you continue to pay the Medicare Part B monthly premium of $42.50.

Many beneficiaries find that coordinated care plans are a good way to get more health care for their dollar. HMOs provide or arrange for all Medicare-covered services and generally charge a fixed monthly premium and small copayments. This makes out-of-pocket expenses more predictable, and possibly minimizes these expenses.

Coordinated plans may also offer benefits not covered by Medicare for little or no additional cost to the beneficiary. Benefits can include preventive care, dental care, hearing aids, eyeglasses, prescription drugs, chiropractic care, and other benefits.

Enrollment

Most Medicare beneficiaries are eligible to enroll in managed care plans. Since most managed care plans available are risk contracts, this section addresses enrollment for these plans.

Plans cannot screen their applicants to find whether they are healthy, or delay coverage for pre-existing conditions (see next section for exceptions). The only enrollment criteria for Medicare managed care plans are:

- The beneficiary must be enrolled in Part B and continue to pay Part B premiums. (Eligibility for Part A is not a factor.)

- The beneficiary must live in the plan's service area.

- The beneficiary cannot be receiving care in a Medicare-certified hospice.

- The beneficiary cannot have permanent kidney failure.

If the beneficiary develops permanent kidney failure or chooses hospice coverage after joining the HMO, the plan is to provide, pay for, or arrange for care. Plans must hold an open enrollment period of at least 30 days at least once per year. Beneficiaries can enroll at this time and may dis-enroll by providing written notice, which will remove the beneficiary from the rolls by the end of the month in which the notice is received. Should you enroll in a plan and later move out of the plan's service area or otherwise choose to discontinue, you can either return to standard fee-for-service Medicare or enroll in another plan for your new location.

Types of Managed Care Plans

Medicare has three types of contracts with managed care plans: *risk* contracts, *cost* contracts, and *health care prepayment plan* (HCPP) agreements. It is important to understand the differences among the three because the type of contract the plan has with Medicare affects the type of coverage you will receive. Before signing with a managed care plan, you may want to find out what type of contract the plan has with HCFA.

Risk contracts refer to plans that agree to accept the financial risk of insuring and caring for a Medicare beneficiary. Most plans are risk contract plans. Cost contract plans, as the name implies, interact with the Medicare program based on the cost of providing services. All risk and cost contract plans must provide all of the Medicare benefits generally available in the plan's service area.

Whether you are entitled to Parts A and B, or Part B only, you can get all of your Medicare benefits through the plan. Both of these types of plans may also offer extra benefits, not otherwise covered by Medicare. Some of these extra benefits include physicals and other preventive care, prescription drugs, dental care, hearing aids, eyeglasses, and foreign travel coverage.

Risk contract plans may provide the extra benefits at no additional cost to you or they can require you to purchase them as a condition of enrolling in the plan. Cost plans are *not* permitted to provide extra benefits at no cost and *cannot* require you to purchase extra benefits.

Risk contract plans also have "lock-in" requirements, which means that the enrollee is locked into receiving all covered care through the plan or through referrals by the plan. If you go outside the plan for services, neither the plan nor Medicare will pay for those services. You will be liable for payment of the entire bill. Exceptions to this rule are for emergency services, which you may receive anywhere in the United States, and urgently needed care, which you may receive while temporarily away from the plan's service area.

Cost contract plans do not have lock-in requirements. This means you can either go to providers affiliated with the plan and pay only the plan's applicable copayments, or you can go outside the plan. If you go outside the plan, Medicare pays its share of the approved charges, just as it does under standard fee-for-service, and you are responsible for applicable deductible and coinsurance amounts, plus any amounts in excess of the Medicare-approved amount.

HCPP agreement plans are a little different. A plan with a HCPP agreement may provide you with services in the same general manner as under a cost contract and, like a cost plan, you are not locked into receiving services from the plan's providers. However, HCPP plans do not have to offer the full range of Medicare benefits nor do they have to comply with all the requirements that apply to cost and risk plans.

For example, HCPP plans are not required to offer an open enrollment period and the plan can refuse to enroll you based on the status of your health. In addition, the Medicare rules that do apply only affect payment for services covered by Part B. If the plan provides Part A services for a prepaid amount that covers Medicare deductibles and coinsurance, that part of your arrangement with the plan is not governed by Medicare rules.

WHICH INSURANCE SHOULD I CHOOSE?

Medicare beneficiaries have quite a few choices for coverage. How should you choose? Choose the option that works best for *you*. This may not be the same plan your best friend, your neighbor, or your colleague chooses, but it should be the best for you and your needs. Some coverage options you have include:

Fee-for-service Medicare and a Medigap policy. This option provides you with the greatest choice in doctors and hospitals, some protection from liability for emergency services if you travel temporarily outside the United States, and coverage for most illnesses you may contract. This option does not provide long-term or custodial care, but you could purchase an additional policy to cover nursing home care. A disadvantage of this option could be the cost, since a Medigap policy can run as high as $150 per month. Coupled with the Medicare Part B premium at $42.50, this makes your monthly expense for health insurance almost $200.

Fee-for-service Medicare and retiree coverage. The difference between this option and the option above is the coverage "secondary" to Medicare. That is, Medigap policies and their benefits are standardized and are usually purchased by the beneficiary. Retiree coverage, on the other hand, is coverage available to a beneficiary upon his retirement from work. Often, retiree coverage is provided at no or very little cost to the retiree, and sometimes provides benefits that Medigap policies do not provide, such as prescription drug coverage or payment for dental services. In addition, the beneficiary usually has no waiting period or exclusions for preexisting conditions. However, retiree coverage is not a Medigap plan and is not regulated. This means the plan may not supplement Medicare benefits in the same way a Medigap plan does.

Until recently, it was unlawful for a Medigap insurer to sell you a Medigap plan if you also had retiree coverage. This is no longer true. You can purchase a Medigap plan even if it duplicates your retiree coverage, and the Medigap plan must pay full benefits even if the retiree plan also pays for the same services. However, if the retiree plan contains a coordination of benefits clause, it may not pay duplicate benefits. While purchasing a Medigap policy in addition to your retiree coverage would "cover all bases," it may also be an unnecessary expense. Read your retiree plan benefits carefully to determine whether a Medigap plan in addition to this plan is truly warranted.

Managed care. Managed care can be a very good option for some seniors. It offers the advantage of no Medicare deductibles and copayments and, very often, offers benefits beyond what Medicare provides for very little additional cost. As long as you do not travel far from home very often, this option can be quite advantageous. Also, many beneficiaries appreciate managed care because no paperwork is required from them; no claim forms to file, no additional insurance company to deal with, etc. (The same is true of most Medigap plans.) However, some beneficiaries do not like the managed care option because their choice of doctors is restricted. But, if your doctor is part of the Medicare managed care plan, you may want to consider this option, especially if additional benefits for little additional cost are provided.

Employer group health plan and delayed Medicare enrollment. For those beneficiaries who continue to work after age 65, the choice of whether to accept the employer's group health plan and delay enrollment in Medicare Part B or to decline the employer's coverage and select Medicare coverage can be a difficult one. The two most important factors to consider in this choice are price and coverage. If the employer plan costs little more than Medicare but covers many more services, you should probably consider delaying enrollment in Medicare Part B. (Your Medigap mandatory acceptance provision is protected because it activates when you enroll in Medicare Part B, not when you are eligible.) However, if the employer plan does not offer any additional benefits or is more expensive, you may want to consider Medicare coverage. This decision can be difficult and should be well thought out. The following should help you make this choice.

Choosing Between an Employer's Group Health Plan and Medicare

Beneficiaries have the option of choosing Medicare benefits or those offered by their employer (or spouse's employer). While it is always nice to have a choice, it is important to know the consequences of each choice. First, if you reject the group health plan, the plan *cannot* offer to pay for any Medicare-covered services or offer to buy or sponsor supplemental coverage. However, the plan *can* offer insurance for services that are not covered by Medicare, such as hearing aids and dental services.

To determine whether you should accept or reject the employer plan, you need to evaluate what benefits are provided and at what cost. Medicare Part A and Part B cover a wide range of services for relatively low cost (no premium for Part A, $42.50 per month for Part B). Accepting Part A coverage is not an issue; it costs nothing and your entitlement is automatic (unless you have not applied for Social Security benefits). If you delay enrollment, you may be required to pay a penalty in the form of a premium, so enroll for Part A coverage. Medicare will pay secondary to your employer plan as long as the plan is in effect (see Chapter Nine for more on Medicare as secondary payer).

Accepting Part B coverage requires more deliberation. Medicare Part B does not cover some items routinely needed by seniors, such as hearing aids, eye glasses, prescription drugs, routine dental care, and an annual physical examination. If your employer plan does offer these items in addition to those covered by Medicare for a cost not much higher than Medicare's, you may want to consider accepting the employer plan.

To illustrate how one might make this decision, consider an example. Mrs. Middleton, now 64, has group health insurance through her employer. But she will be turning 65 soon and she is trying to decide whether she should terminate this coverage in favor of Medicare coverage. To make this decision, she must first identify what services she receives each year and at what cost.

Mrs. Middleton has her teeth cleaned twice a year at a cost of $80 each visit ($160 per year), sees her internist once a year for a routine physical ($105) and pap smear ($40), sees her internist four times a year to monitor her high blood pressure at a cost of $60 per visit ($240 annually), and takes medication for the high blood pressure at a cost of $33 per month ($396 per year). Her total bill for health care services is $941 per year.

Group health plan

The monthly premium for the group health plan is $115, of which Mrs. Middleton only pays 20 percent, or $23 per month. This plan does not pay for her routine physical and pap smear or routine dental services, but does pay for her blood pressure medication as a regular claim. The group health plan has an annual deductible of $250 and coinsurance of 20 percent of the usual, customary, and reasonable charge (which is the charge her internist makes). So, under the group health plan, Mrs. Middleton will pay:

Monthly premium ($ 23 x 12 months)	**$276.00**
Noncovered services (dental cleanings, routine physical, pap smear)	**$305.00**
Deductible	**$250.00**
Coinsurance	**$ 77.20**
January visit	$ 60.00
January medication	$ 33.00
February medication	$ 33.00

March medication	$ 33.00
April visit	$ 60.00
April medication	$ 33.00
Deductible satisfied	
May medication	$ 33.00
June medication	$ 33.00
July visit	$ 60.00
July medication	$ 33.00
August medication	$ 33.00
September medication	$ 33.00
October visit	$ 60.00
October medication	$ 33.00
November medication	$ 33.00
December medication	$ 33.00
Total after deductible was satisfied **($386 x .20) =**	$77.20

Total costs =   **$908.20**

$276 (premium) + $305 (noncovered services) + $250 (deductible) + $77.20 (coinsurance) = $ 908.20

Medicare

Mrs. Middleton would be responsible for Part B premiums of $42.50 per month. Medicare would not pay for her routine dental services or routine physical, but would pay for the pap smear. Medicare also would not pay for her blood pressure medication. Medicare's annual deductible is $100 and coinsurance is 20 percent of Medicare's allowable, which is lower than the usual, customary and reasonable charge. (Mrs. Middleton obtained this information by contacting the local carrier.) So, Mrs. Middleton will pay:

Monthly premium ($42.50 x 12 months)	**$510.00**
Noncovered services (dental cleanings, routine physical, medication)	**$676.00**
Deductible	**$100.00**
Coinsurance	**$ 16.00**
January visit	$ 40.00
Pap smear	$ 20.00
April visit	$ 40.00

Deductible satisfied

July visit	$ 40.00
October visit	$ 40.00

Total after deductible
was satisfied (**$ 80.00 x .20**) = $ 16.00

Total costs = **$1,302.00**

$510.00 (premiums) + $676.00 (noncovered services) + $100.00 (deductible) + $16.00 (coinsurance) = $1302.00

The difference is $393.80 in favor of the employer plan.

Mrs. Middleton decided to accept the employer plan, with the stipulation that she would reevaluate in one year.

Other Factors to Consider When Choosing Additional Insurance

Shop carefully. Policies differ in coverage and cost, and companies differ in quality and service. Compare companies and plans carefully. The following tips should help you make an appropriate choice.

• In evaluating a policy, check for preexisting condition waiting periods and exclusions. If you have a health problem, the insurer may not cover expenses related to treatment of that condition, either permanently or for a limited period of time. (Medigap policies are required to cover preexisting conditions after the policy has been in effect for six months.)

• Be aware of maximum benefits where the policy restricts either the dollar amount that will be paid for treatment of a condition or the number of days of care for which payment will be made. Some employer policies pay less than the Medicare allowable for hospital outpatient medical services and for services provided in a physician's office. Others do not pay anything toward the cost of these services. Read the policy and be aware of what it will actually pay for and in what amount.

• Don't buy more insurance than you need. A single comprehensive policy is better than several policies with overlapping or duplicate coverage. (The law prohibits insurers from selling you a second Medigap policy unless you state in writing that you intend to cancel your existing policy and replace it with the new policy.) Determine your needs and make a choice based on those needs. Remember, the more policies you have, the more complicated it will be to determine who should pay and when.

- Be familiar with the agent and the company with whom you intend to deal. You can check with your state's insurance commission to see if the company is licensed to do business in your state. Agents must also be licensed by the state and may be required by the state to carry proof of licensure. A business card is not a license; check with the insurance commission or company the agent claims to represent if you are unsure about his sincerity. Also, write down the agent's name and phone number and the company's name, phone number, and address. If you have a problem or a question, this information will be necessary.

- Take your time. Don't let an agent pressure you into buying. There is no legitimate reason for making a snap decision about your health insurance. The only time constraint you need to consider is the six-month open enrollment period for Medigap plans where no special conditions for your insurance can be imposed.

- When you do decide to purchase, complete the application carefully. Failure to include requested information can cause the insurer to exclude certain conditions from coverage or deny or revoke your coverage altogether. Whether intentional or not, a material misrepresentation of the facts is grounds for denial of an application or revocation of a policy currently in force. Take your time and obtain the necessary information.

- Always use a check or money order, payable to the insurance company (not the agent), to pay your premium. Do not use cash. Get a receipt for your payment that includes the company's name, address, and telephone number, and keep it with your copy of your application and other relevant documents.

- When you receive your summary of the insurance policy, read it carefully. If something does not make sense or seems contrary to what the agent told you, ask. If the agent does not answer your questions to your satisfaction, call the company directly. If the policy is a Medigap plan, you have 30 days to review it and cancel if you don't like it. Use this time wisely.

CHAPTER 6

THE APPEALS PROCESS
FOR PART A

The appeals process offers an opportunity to "contest" the determination made by a carrier or intermediary on a particular claim. If you don't like the determination made on your claim, you have recourse—you're not "stuck" with it.

Unfortunately, many beneficiaries believe they either cannot appeal a determination, or that it is too difficult to do so. Also, many believe that the determination will not be changed anyway, "so why bother?" This is simply not true!

Part A decisions are reversed or overturned on appeal almost half of the time. Approximately two out of three Part B decisions are reversed at the first level of appeal. It can be well worth your time to request an appeal.

The procedures for appealing a decision for a Part A differ from those for a Part B claim. To help you understand the differences and improve your chances for a successful appeal, this chapter provides information about the appeals process for Part A. The next chapter is devoted to the appeals process for Part B.

In either case, there are three terms that deserve special definition as they pertain to the appeals process:

A *determination* is the decision made by either a carrier, an intermediary, or in the case of hospital inpatient services, a Peer Review Organization (PRO), to pay or deny all or part of the services billed on a particular claim.

Decisions are made by providers regarding possible coverage of Medicare services; they are not official Medicare determinations and cannot be appealed. It is important to distinguish between a determination and a decision. Only a Medicare contractor can make a determination and only determinations can be appealed. The beneficiary, his representative, or a physician can appeal a determination.

The person who files the appeal is referred to as the *claimant*.

GENERAL PRINCIPLES

The appeals process for Part A claims consists of three levels: the reconsideration, the administrative law judge (ALJ) hearing, and the Appeals Council hearing. An appeal must start at the lowest level—the reconsideration—and proceed "upward." This means that if you are dissatisfied with the reconsideration determination, you move to the next level. You cannot immediately request an Appeals Council hearing if you have not had a reconsideration and an ALJ hearing first.

Part A services are adjudicated by either a Peer Review Organization (PRO) or the intermediary. Intermediaries make determinations and payment for skilled nursing facility (SNF), home health agency, and hospice care. Services furnished by these providers are first appealed to the intermediary.

PROs make determinations for hospital inpatient services. (The PRO does not issue payment; the intermediary makes the actual payment to the provider pursuant to the PRO's determination.)

The PRO's chief function is to ensure the medical necessity, quality, and appropriateness of hospital care provided to Medicare beneficiaries. PROs have authority to deny Medicare payment for inappropriate or unnecessary services. They can also recommend exclusion from the

Medicare program for utilization patterns and practices of providers and physicians. Inappropriate care refers to the appropriateness of admissions, i.e., does the patient's condition require hospitalization? Necessity of services refers to the length of stay, i.e., does the patient need continued hospitalization based on his condition?

The Social Security Act also defines another responsibility of the PRO: to monitor the performance of hospitals under the Prospective Payment System (PPS). Specifically, to review and determine: "the validity of diagnostic information provided by a hospital; the completeness, adequacy, and quality of care provided; the appropriateness of admissions and discharges; and the appropriateness of care for which additional payment is sought" (Section 1866(a)(1)(M) of the Act). Hospital services are first appealed to the PRO.

The process of obtaining a determination and appealing it can be quite involved. While a successful appeal is possible on your own, it is advisable that you seek the advice of a professional advocate, such as an attorney or beneficiary advocacy organization, to help with your appeal.

The advocate should be knowledgeable about Medicare regulations and rulings, and have experience with the Medicare Part A appeals process. The advocate will complete this process for you, and will probably be more efficient and effective because of his experience. Should you decide to appoint an advocate to represent you in an appeal, you will need to notify Medicare of your decision. To do this, you must file a completed Form SSA-1696-U4 "Appointment of Representative." A copy of the form is shown in Figure 6-1.

Figure 6-1: Form SSA-1696-U4, Appointment of Representative

DEPARTMENT OF
HEALTH AND HUMAN SERVICES
HEALTH CARE FINANCING ADMINISTRATION

NAME (Print or Type)	H.I. Claim Number

Section I   **APPOINTMENT OF REPRESENTATIVE**

I appoint this individual: _____
(Print or type name and address of individual you want to represent you.)
to act as my representative in connection with my claim or asserted right under Titles XI, or XVIII of the Social Security Act. I authorize this individual to make or give any request or notice; to present or to elicit evidence; to obtain information; and to receive any notice in connection with my claim wholly in my stead.

SIGNATURE (Beneficiary)	ADDRESSS
TELEPHONE NUMBER (Area Code)	DATE

Section II   **ACCEPTANCE OF APPOINTMENT**

I, _____, hereby accept the above appointment. I certify that I have not been suspended or prohibited from practice before the Social Security Administration or the Health Care Financing Administration; that I am not, as a current or former officer or employee of the United States, disqualified from acting as the claimant's representative; and that I will not charge or receive any fee for the representation unless it has been authorized in accordance with the laws and regulations referred to on the reverse side hereof. In the event that I decide not to charge or collect a fee for the representation I will notify the Social Security Administration and the Health Care Financing Administration (completion of Section III (optional) satisfies this requirement).

I am a / an _____
(Attorney, union representative, relative, law student, etc.)

SIGNATURE (Representative)	ADDRESS
TELEPHONE NUMBER (Area Code)	DATE

Section III (Optional)   **WAIVER OF FEE OR DIRECT PAYMENT**

(Note to Representative: You may use this portion of the form to waive a fee or to waive direct payment of the fee from withheld past-due benefits.)

I waive my right to charge and collect a fee for representing _____
_____ before the Social Security Administration or Health Care Financing Administration.

SIGNATURE	DATE

(See important information on reverse)
Form HCFA-1696-U4 (10-84)   1-FILE COPY

Each level of appeal has two requirements: a time limit within which the appeal must be filed and a minimum dollar amount in question (also called the "amount in controversy"). The charts shown in Figures 6-2 and 6-3 illustrate the time and amount in controversy limits for Part A appeals.

To meet the amount in controversy requirement, you may combine claims that have been reconsidered if all claims combined have been reconsidered by the intermediary and you want a hearing on them and the request for hearing is filed on time for each claim in the request. The amount in controversy minimum does not have to be reached with a single claim, and two or more people may combine reconsidered claims if the combined claims were denied for the same reason.

The time limit for filing an appeal can be extended if the you can show good cause why you did not file within the time limit. Examples of conditions that establish good cause are:

- Mental or physical impairment (e.g., disability or extended illness) or significant communication difficulties.

- Advanced age or death.

- Incorrect or incomplete information regarding the claim in question provided by official sources, such as HCFA or the carrier.

- Delay in securing supporting evidence where the individual did not know that evidence could be submitted after filing.

Figure 6-2: Medicare Part A Appeals—Hospital Care

Stage of Appeal:	Reconsideration Request	Hearing Request	Request for Appeals Council Review	Request For Judicial Review
Time Deadline for Filing Appeal:	60 days after Notice of Medicare Claim Determination (or within 3 days if request expedited appeal)	60 days after Reconsideration determination	60 days after Hearing decision	60 days after Appeals Council
Amount of Claim:	No minimum	$200 minimum*	$200 minimum*	$2,000 min.*
File Appeal Request With:	Hospital's PRO or local Social Security office	Hospital's PRO processed and forwarded to Social Security Office of Hearings and Appeals, or local Social Security office	Social Security's Appeals Council	United States District Court
Appeal Reviewed and Decided By:	Hospital's PRO	Social Security Office of Hearings and Appeals	Social Security's Appeals Council	United States District Court
Time Deadline For Decision:	3 days if inpatient or preadmission; 30 days for all others	None	None	None

*If the appeal is on a question of entitlement to Part A benefits, there is no minimum amount required.

Figure 6-2 is reproduced with permission from the Legal Counsel for the Elderly, *Medicare Practice Manual* © 1990.

Figure 6-3: Medicare Part A Appeals—Skilled Nursing Facility, Home Health, and Hospice Care

Stage of Appeal:	Reconsideration Request	Hearing Request	Request for Appeals Council Review	Request for Judicial Review
Time Deadline for Filing Appeal:	60 days after Notice of Medicare Claim Determination or concurrent with patient's written request for payment	60 days after Reconsideration determination	60 days after Hearing decision	60 days after Appeals Council
Amount of Claim:	No minimum	$100 minimum*	$100 minimum*	$1,000 min.*
File Appeal Request With:	Skilled nursing facility's or home health agency's intermediary, or local Social Security office	Skilled nursing facility's or home health agency's intermediary (processed and forwarded to Social Security Office of Hearings and Appeals) or local Social Security Office	Social Security Appeals Council	United States District Court
Appeal Reviewed and Decided By:	Intermediary from Social Security	Administrative law judge Social Security's Office of Hearings and Appeals	Social Security Appeals Council	United States District Court

*If the appeal is on a questions of entitlement to Part A benefits, there is no minimum amount required.

Figure 6-3 is reproduced with permission from the Legal Counsel for the Elderly, *Medicare Practice Manual* © 1990.

- Destruction or damage of records, such as in a fire or flood.

TYPES OF DENIALS

Before discussing the process of appealing a determination, it's helpful to first understand the types of typical denial decisions. Admission denials are those that occur because the hospital is unsure about Medicare coverage of the admission based on the patient's condition. This typically occurs because coverage for the same condition has previously been denied for other patients. Because the hospital will not be paid for services unless the beneficiary is aware that Medicare will not cover the services, often the hospital denies admittance or asks the beneficiary to bear the financial burden associated with his care.

The other type of denial is where the medical necessity of the patient's length of stay is being questioned. Premature discharges occur because the hospital has a financial incentive to limit the amount of time the patient is hospitalized. Recall that hospitals are paid a predetermined amount based on the patient's diagnosis. The longer the patient is in the hospital, the more it costs to care for him. Discharge at the earliest possible time maximizes the hospital's profit and minimizes the hospital's loss associated with that patient.

HOSPITAL INPATIENT SERVICES

When you are admitted to a hospital, you are provided with a copy of a notice called "Your Rights as a Medicare Hospital Inpatient" (see Figure 2-2 in Chapter Two). This form contains information related to appealing decisions and determinations. Read this, keep it with you or give it to a family member. Refer to it if you have a question. It will help explain what to do if you don't agree with a hospital's decision or if you wish to appeal a determination.

All hospitals are required by law to have a utilization review committee (URC). These review the medical necessity of hospital admissions and the duration of hospital stays. At least two members of the URC must be physicians.

Before deciding that a hospital admission or longer stay is not medically necessary, the URC must talk with the doctor responsible for the particular patient's care. The committee must give him an opportunity to present his views regarding the necessity of admission or continued stay.

If the URC decides that coverage will be denied because the admission or continued stay is unnecessary, it must provide written notice to the hospital, the patient, and the attending physician. The hospital provides the patient with a notice of noncoverage, which informs him of the hospital's decision. A sample notice is shown in Figure 2-1 in Chapter Two.

A notice of noncoverage is a statement of the *decision made by the hospital*; you cannot appeal it to Medicare. However, if you disagree with the hospital's decision and want to remain in the hospital, note the date and time the notice was received. Then, submit a written request for a review to the PRO in your state. Make your request immediately because your stay in the hospital is covered for only two additional days after the receipt of the discharge notice.

The PRO is required to respond to your request within three days. If the PRO approves your continued stay, Medicare will cover the additional days. If the PRO does not approve the continuation, you will have to pay all hospital costs beginning on the third day after receipt of the notice of noncoverage.

If the hospital is denying admission because it believes Medicare will not pay, the hospital must notify you of this in writing. If you disagree with the hospital, you can ask that the PRO provide an official determination. You must request the determination within 30 days of the hospital's decision. Or you can ask for an expedited determination, which means the PRO will issue a determination within three days. You can make this request to the PRO in writing or by telephone, but in either case the request must be made within three days of the date you received the hospital's decision.

If the PRO decides coverage is available, the hospital should admit you. If the PRO denies coverage, then the hospital is not obligated to admit you. Or, if the hospital does allow you to be admitted, it will be with the understanding that Medicare will not pay—so you will be expected to.

The beneficiary must be provided with advance written notice informing him that Medicare will not pay for a service because it is not medically necessary. Failure to provide the beneficiary with this notice forfeits the provider's right to collect payment for the services. (See also the discussion of limitation of liability.)

The notice of noncoverage protects the provider's right to collect payment. The beneficiary's "liability" for payment of the charges is "limited" to paying only for those services that are reasonable and necessary, noncovered, or those for which the beneficiary was aware that Medicare would not pay because they are considered not reasonable and necessary. The chart in Figure 6-4 illustrates the step-by-step process of filing a hospital inpatient appeal.

Figure 6-4: Medicare Hospital Coverage Determination and Appeals Process

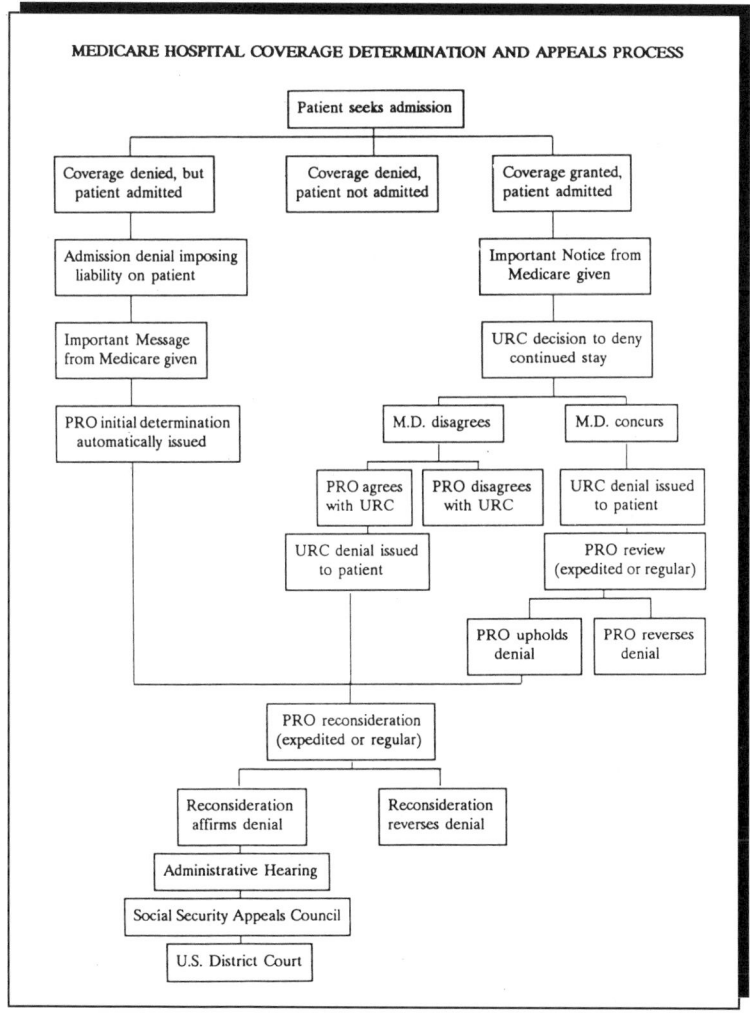

Figure 6-4 is reproduced with permission from The Legal Counsel for the Elderly, *Medicare Practice Manual*, 1990. The discussion following is adapted from the *Medicare Practice Manual* as well.

The determination and appeals process depicted in Figure 6-4 works like this:

1. The patient comes to the hospital seeking admission, usually on the advice of a physician.

2. When patient seeks admission, a hospital may choose one of three courses of action:

   • Decide the patient will be covered by Medicare and admit the patient.

   • Decide Medicare coverage is not available but permit the patient to enter the hospital anyway. The hospital will usually issue the patient a notice of admission denial, informing him that the cost of hospital care will be his responsibility.

   • Deny Medicare coverage and not admit the patient. Often the patient will balk at assuming responsibility for expensive care and the hospital may simply refuse to allow the patient to enter. Usually no written Medicare denial notice is issued, and the patient has no right to appeal. An exception exists, however, where the PRO has a preadmission review process in place.

     Although unusual, involvement of the PRO at the preadmission stage is good because appeal is then possible. In such cases, the PRO reviews the medical necessity or appropriateness of some or all of the Medicare admissions before they occur.

If the PRO determines that Medicare coverage is not available, it issues an initial determination notice to the beneficiary. It is this initial determination than can be appealed.

3. All patients actually admitted to the hospital must be given a special notice called "An Important Message From Medicare." (A copy is provided in Figure 2-2.) This mandatory notice is very explicit about a patient's rights while in the hospital. Most of the information in this notice concerns the procedure to be followed when the hospital issues a continuing care denial of Medicare coverage. A continuing care denial occurs when the patient has been granted Medicare coverage on admission, but the hospital, usually acting through its Utilization Review Committee, decides that the patient no longer needs a hospital level of care.

4. Utilization review of a continued stay usually occurs because the stay needed is longer or more expensive than the average for that diagnostic related group (DRG). (Refer to Chapter Four for more information about payment methodology.) Before issuing a decision that an admission or a continued stay is not medically necessary, the Utilization Review Committee must consult the attending physician and give him an opportunity to present his point of view.

5. The hospital's principal motivation when such a case has been identified is to avoid the financial loss represented by the gap between the DRG payment and the cost of the patient's care as the stay continues. Before a hospital may bill a patient for the cost of services provided, however, the hospital must comply

with a complex coverage determination, notice, and appeals process.

Federal regulations are quite specific concerning when a hospital may charge a Medicare patient for hospital services. Generally, a hospital may not charge a beneficiary for any service for which payment is made by Medicare, even if the hospital's cost of furnishing services to the patient is greater than the amount the hospital is paid under PPS. The hospital is always permitted to charge the patient the applicable deductible and coinsurance amounts. The hospital is not permitted to charge the patient for care excluded from Medicare coverage, as custodial care or medically unnecessary care, unless the following specific steps are followed:

- The hospital must decide that the patient no longer requires inpatient hospital care. This includes cases where a beneficiary needs SNF-level care but, under Medicare criteria, that level bed is not available.

- If the attending physician agrees with the hospital's decision in writing, the hospital may immediately issue a continuing care denial to the patient. If the attending physician believes that hospital-level care is still required, the hospital may request an immediate review of the case by the PRO. Concurrence by the PRO with the hospital's decision serves in lieu of the physician's agreement, and the denial notice may then be given to the patient.

- The continuing care denial notice given to the patient must inform the patient that customary charges will be assessed against him only after the *second day following the date of the notice.* For example, if a patient receives a denial notice on Monday, the patient may not be charged for the cost of care until Thursday.

  For a case where coverage is denied on admission and no covered days are granted, the hospital may not charge the patient for hospital care that is not medically necessary until the patient has been notified in writing that Medicare coverage is not available. The notice must also inform the patient concerning the appeal rights described below.

6. The right to appeal for a patient given a continuing care denial differs depending on whether the attending physician concurred with the URC's denial decision or whether the URC was required to obtain PRO approval of the proposed determination.

   If the attending physician agreed with the hospital's decision of noncoverage, the PRO was not required to review the case. In this situation the patient is entitled to an expedited PRO review. If the patient is still an inpatient in the hospital and requests an expedited review, it should take place no later than noon of the first working day after the date the patient receives the URC denial notice.

   The hospital is required to provide the PRO with a copy of the medical records by the close of business on that working day, and the PRO must issue a determination not later than one full working day after the date the PRO received the request for expedited review and the medical records. The hospital may not charge the patient for inpatient hospital services after the date the patient or representative receives notice of the PRO's expedited decision. If the patient is no longer in the hospital, or fails to request an expedited determination on time, the PRO is required to issue a determination within 30 days of the request.

If the patient's attending physician does not concur with the hospital's decision of noncoverage, the hospital must obtain the PRO's concurrence before it can bill the patient. The PRO must give an opportunity to the provider and to the physician to discuss the merits of the case.

If the PRO concurs with the hospital's decision, the hospital is informed by the PRO and the hospital will issue a notice to the patient. The PRO's concurrence constitutes an initial determination, and the PRO will also issue a notice to the patient. In cases where the hospital has sought and received the PRO's agreement, the appropriate appeal is for reconsideration rather than review (because the PRO has already reviewed the case).

If the beneficiary is still an inpatient when the PRO receives a request for reconsideration, the PRO must complete its determination and send a notice to the beneficiary within three working days after the PRO receives the reconsideration request. If the beneficiary is no longer a hospital inpatient, the PRO must issue the reconsideration decision within 30 working days.

It is unclear to what extent a hospital is required to notify the family members or legal representative of ill or incompetent patients. In one case, the court found that the hospital had a duty to provide written, not oral, notice of the denial of Medicare coverage to the friend of an incompetent patient, where the hospital knew that the friend was acting on the patient's behalf. In practice, hospitals usually attempt to notify both the patient and the relative or representative who has been acting on the patient's behalf.

7. The patient may appeal the PRO's initial determination by requesting a reconsideration. Generally, a dissatisfied party must file a request for reconsideration within 60 days after receipt of the notice of the PRO's determination. If the beneficiary is still an inpatient in the hospital when the PRO receives the request for reconsideration, the PRO must complete its reconsideration determination and send written notice to the beneficiary within three working days after the PRO's receipt of the request for reconsideration.

   The PRO must issue the reconsideration determination within 30 working days if the beneficiary is no longer an inpatient in the hospital. A copy of the form used to file the request is shown in Figure 6-5.

8. If the PRO reconsideration is unfavorable, the beneficiary may request a hearing before an administrative law judge (ALJ) of the Social Security Administration's Office of Hearings and Appeals. The amount in controversy must be at least $200. The hearing request must be filed within 60 days of receipt of the notice of the PRO reconsideration determination, unless the time is extended for good cause.

   The request for reconsideration must be filed at the PRO, at a Social Security office, at an SSA Office of Hearings and Appeals, or at an office of the Railroad Retirement Board. A copy of the form used to file the request is shown in Figure 6-6.

Figure 6-5: Form HCFA-2649—Request for Reconsideration of Part A Health Insurance Benefits

DEPARTMENT OF HEALTH AND HUMAN SERVICES
HEALTH CARE FINANCING ADMINISTRATION

Form Approved.
OMB No. 0938-0045

REQUEST FOR RECONSIDERATION OF PART A HEALTH INSURANCE BENEFITS

INSTRUCTIONS: *Please type or print firmly.* Leave the block empty if you cannot answer it. Take or mail the WHOLE form to your Social Security office which will be glad to help you. Please read the statement on the reverse side of page 2.

1. BENEFICIARY'S NAME

2. HEALTH INSURANCE CLAIM NUMBER

3. REPRESENTATIVE'S NAME, IF APPLICABLE
☐ RELATIVE ☐ ATTORNEY ☐ OTHER PERSON) ☐ PROVIDER FILING

4. PLEASE ATTACH A COPY OF THE NOTICE(S) YOU RECEIVED ABOUT YOUR CLAIM TO THIS FORM.

5. THIS CLAIM IS FOR
☐ INPATIENT HOSPITAL ☐ SKILLED NURSING FACILITY (SNF) ☐ HEALTH MAINTENANCE ORGANIZATION (HMO)
☐ EMERGENCY HOSPITAL ☐ HOME HEALTH AGENCY (HHA)

6. NAME AND ADDRESS OF PROVIDER (Hospital, SNF, HHA, HMO)

CITY AND STATE

PROVIDER NUMBER

7. NAME OF INTERMEDIARY

CITY AND STATE

INTERMEDIARY NUMBER

8. DATE OF ADMISSON OR START OF SERVICES

9. DATE(S) OF THE NOTICE(S) YOU RECEIVED

10. I DO NOT AGREE WITH THE DETERMINATION ON MY CLAIM. PLEASE RECONSIDER MY CLAIM BECAUSE

11. YOU MUST OBTAIN ANY EVIDENCE (For example, a letter from a doctor) YOU WISH TO SUBMIT

☐ I HAVE ATTACHED THE FOLLOWING EVIDENCE

☐ I WILL SEND THIS EVIDENCE WITHIN 10 DAYS

☐ I HAVE NO ADDITIONAL EVIDENCE OR OTHER INFORMATION TO SUBMIT WITH MY CLAIM

13. ONLY ONE SIGNATURE IS NEEDED. THIS FORM IS SIGNED BY
☐ BENEFICIARY ☐ REPRESENTATIVE ☐ PROVIDER REP

SIGN HERE ▶

14. STREET ADDRESS

12. IS THIS REQUEST FILED WITHIN 60 DAYS OF THE DATE OF YOUR NOTICE?
☐ YES ☐ NO
IF YOU CHECKED "NO" ATTACH AN EXPLANATION OF THE REASON FOR THE DELAY TO THIS FORM

CITY, STATE, ZIP CODE

TELEPHONE

DATE

15. If this request is signed by mark (X), TWO WITNESSES who know the person requesting reconsideration must sign in the space provided on the reverse side of this page of the form.

DO NOT FILL IN BELOW THIS LINE—FOR SOCIAL SECURITY USE—THANK YOU

16. ROUTING
☐ INTERMEDIARY
☐ HCFA RO-MEDICARE
☐ BSS ODR

18. SSA OR INTERMEDIARY DATE STAMP

17. ADDITIONAL INFORMATION

FORM **HCFA-2649** (8-79)
DESTROY PRIOR EDITIONS

INTERMEDIARY FILE

Figure 6-6: Form HA-5011-U6—Request for Hearing of Part A Health Insurance Benefits

DEPARTMENT OF HEALTH AND HUMAN SERVICES
HEALTH CARE FINANCING ADMINISTRATION

REQUEST FOR HEARING
HOSPITAL INSURANCE BENEFITS PAYABLE UNDER **PART A** OF TITLE XVIII
(Amount in Controversy, $100.00 or more)
Take or mail original and all copies to your local Social Security office

SEE PRIVACY ACT NOTICE ON REVERSE SIDE OF FORM.

CLAIMANT

WAGE EARNER (Leave blank if same as above)

HI CLAIM NUMBER

NAME AND ADDRESS OF INTERMEDIARY OR PROFESSIONAL STANDARDS REVIEW ORGANIZATION

CLAIM FOR
☐ Inpatient Hospital Services
☐ Skilled Nursing Facility Services
☐ Home Health Agency Services
☐ Emergency Services
☐ Other (Identify)

PERIOD IN QUESTION
FROM   TO
NAME AND ADDRESS OF PROVIDER (INSTITUTION)

I disagree with the determination made on the above claim and request a hearing. My reasons for disagreement are

Check ONLY ONE of the statements below
☐ I have additional evidence to submit (Attach such evidence to this form or forward to the Social Security Office within 10 days.)

☐ I have no additional evidence to submit.

Check ONLY ONE of the statements below
☐ I wish to appear in person.

☐ I do not wish to appear at a hearing. I request that a decision be made on the basis of the evidence in my case.

Signed by (Either the claimant or representative should sign — Enter addresses for both. If claimant has a representative, Form SSA-1696-U3 (Appointment of Representative) must be completed.)

SIGNATURE OR NAME OF CLAIMANT'S REPRESENTATIVE ☐ Attorney ☐ Non-Attorney

CLAIMANT'S SIGNATURE

ADDRESS

ADDRESS

CITY, STATE, AND ZIP CODE

CITY, STATE, AND ZIP CODE

AREA CODE AND TELEPHONE NUMBER   DATE

AREA CODE AND TELEPHONE NUMBER

Claimant should not fill in below this line

TO BE COMPLETED BY SOCIAL SECURITY ADMINISTRATION

Is this request timely filed? ☐ YES ☐ No
If "No" is checked: (1) Attach claimant's explanation for delay. (2) Attach any pertinent letter, material, or information in the Social Security Office

Interpreter Needed _____
(Language, including sign language)

ACKNOWLEDGMENT OF REQUEST FOR HEARING
This request for hearing was filed on _____ at _____
The Administrative Law Judge will notify you of the time and place of the hearing at least 10 days in advance of the hearing.

HEARING OFFICE COPY

TO
☐ Hearing Office _____
(Location)

For the Social Security Administration
By _____
(Signature)

CLAIM FILE COPY

TO
☐ HCFA, Bureau of Program Operations
Attn. Recon and Eval Branch
Box 770, Baltimore, Md. 21203

☐ HCFA, Medicare Bureau
Regional Office _____

(Title)

(Street Address)

(City, State, and Zip Code)

Servicing Social Security Office Code _____

Form **HA-5011-U6** (10-82)
7/81 edition may be used

ATTACH A COPY OF THE RECONSIDERATION DETERMINATION (IF AVAILABLE) TO THIS COPY

CLAIM FILE

9. If the ALJ hearing is unfavorable, the beneficiary has 60 days to file a request for hearing with the Social Security Administration's Appeals Council in Washington, D.C. The amount in controversy must be at least $1,000. A copy of the form used to file the request is shown in Figure 6-7.

10. Finally, after exhausting administrative appeals, the beneficiary may be able to file a lawsuit in federal court. Certain rules apply to the types of cases that can be heard in federal court; seek the advice and guidance of an attorney, if you have not already.

SKILLED NURSING FACILITY SERVICES

The appeals process for SNF care is not much different than that for hospital inpatient services, except that the appeal is made to the intermediary, rather than a PRO. The chart in Figure 6-8 illustrates the appeals process for SNF services.

Like other areas of Medicare, coverage decisions are made at various levels by a variety of people. Prior to an initial decision by the intermediary, there is an admission decision concerning Medicare coverage made by the SNF. Following Medicare's initial decision, there are three levels of administrative appeal (reconsideration, hearing, Appeals Council hearing) and then judicial review in federal district court.

Figure 6-7: Form HA-520-U5—Request for Review of Hearing Decision

DEPARTMENT OF HEALTH AND HUMAN SERVICES
SOCIAL SECURITY ADMINISTRATION/OFFICE OF HEARINGS AND APPEALS

Form Approved
OMB No. 0960-0277

REQUEST FOR REVIEW OF HEARING DECISION
(Take or mail original and all copies to your local Social Security office)

See Privacy Act
Notice on Reserve

1. CLAIMANT	2. WAGE EARNER, IF DIFFERENT
3. SOCIAL SECURITY CLAIM NUMBER	4. SPOUSE'S NAME AND SOCIAL SECURITY NUMBER. *(Complete ONLY in Supplemental Security Income Case)*

5. I request that the Appeals Council review the Administrative Law Judge's action on the above claim because:

ADDITIONAL EVIDENCE

If you have additional evidence, submit it with this request for review. If you need additional time to submit evidence or legal argument, you must request an extension of time in writing now. If you request an extension of time, you should explain the reason(s) you are unable to submit the evidence or legal argument now. If you neither submit evidence or legal argument now nor within any extension of time the Appeals Council grants, the Appeals Council will take its action based on the evidence of record.

IMPORTANT: Write your Social Security Claim Number on any letter or material you send us.)

SIGNATURE BLOCKS: You should complete No. 6 and your representative (if any) should complete No. 7. If you are represented and your representative is not available to complete this form, you should also print his or her name, address, etc. in No. 7.

DATE	☐ ATTORNEY ☐ NON-ATTORNEY
6. CLAIMANT'S SIGNATURE	7. REPRESENTATIVE'S SIGNATURE
PRINT NAME	PRINT NAME
ADDRESS	ADDRESS
(CITY, STATE, ZIP CODE)	(CITY, STATE, ZIP CODE)
TELEPHONE NUMBER (INCLUDE AREA CODE)	TELEPHONE NUMBER (INCLUDE AREA CODE)

THE SOCIAL SECURITY ADMINISTRATION STAFF WILL COMPLETE THIS PART

8. Request received for the Social Security Administration on _____ by: _____

(Title)	(Address)	Servicing FO Code	PC Code

9. Is the request for review received within 65 days of the ALJ'S Decision/Dismissal? Yes ☐ No ☐

10. If no checked: (1) attach claimant's explanation for delay; and (2) attach copy of appointment notice, letter or other pertinent material or information in the Social Security Office.

11. Check one: ☐ Initial Entitlement ☐ Termination or other	12. Check all claim types that apply:
	☐ Retirement or survivors (RSI)
	☐ Disability—Worker (DIWC)
	☐ Disability—Widow(er) (DIWW)
	☐ Disability—Child (DIWC)
APPEALS COUNCIL OFFICE OF HEARINGS AND APPEALS, SSA 5107 Leesburg Pike FALLS CHURCH, VA 22041 - 3255	☐ SSI Aged (SSIA)
	☐ SSI Blind (SSIB)
	☐ SSI Disability (SSID)
	☐ Health Insurance-Part A (HIA)
	☐ Health Insurance-Part B (HIB)
	☐ Other—Specify: _____

Form HA-520-U5 (3-94)
Destory old stock

CLAIMS FOLDER

Figure 6-8: Medicare Skilled Nursing Facility Claims Submission and Appeals Process

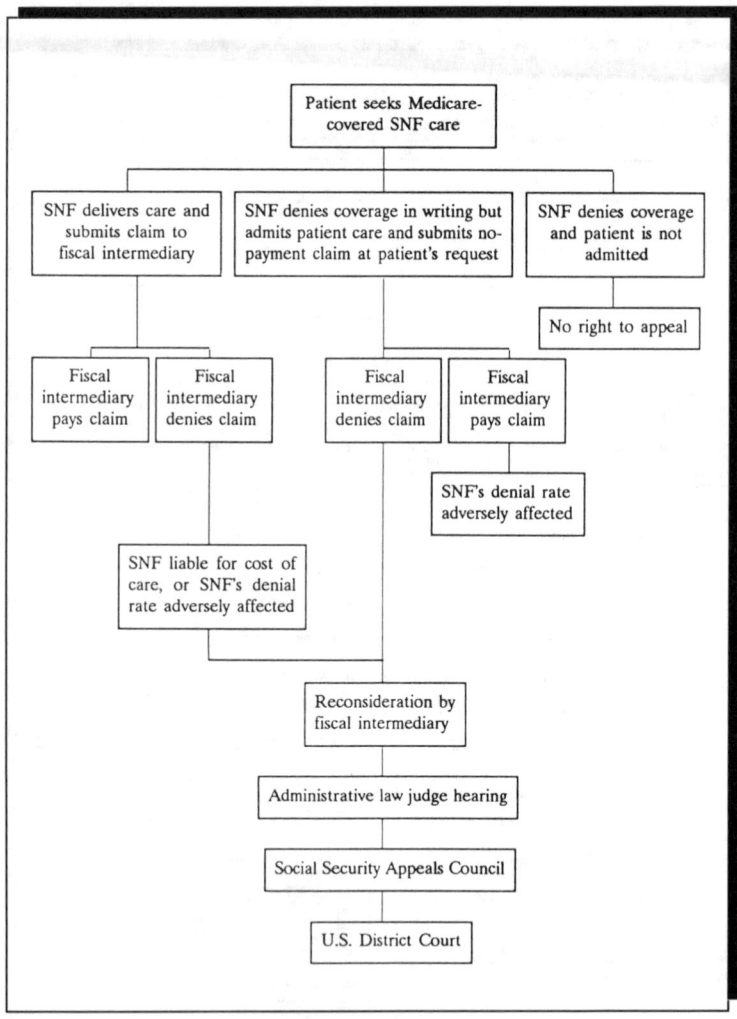

Figure 6-8 is reproduced with permission from the Legal Counsel for the Elderly, *Medicare Practice Manual* © 1990. The discussion following Figure 6-8 was adapted from the *Medicare Practice Manual* as well.

SNF Decisions

Upon transfer from the hospital, the patient is almost always taken to the SNF by ambulance. After arriving at the SNF, the patient is usually taken directly to his room. Necessary paperwork is generally completed by a relative of the patient. (The SNF staff often deal with a relative rather than patients because often patients are unable to fully understand what is going on due to their medical condition).

For the Medicare patient, the most important function of the SNF admission process is the determination that the stay will be covered by Medicare. At the initial stage this critical decision is performed by the SNF. Once admitted to the facility and to a Medicare-certified bed, the patient must have his medical needs assessed to determine whether skilled services are required on a daily basis.

The SNF performs this initial screening process for two reasons. First, the Medicare law and regulations require providers to have in place utilization review plans to ensure that medical services are necessary and that services are being efficiently utilized. As a condition of participation, the provider must perform this function.

Second, the provider is concerned with its "limitation of liability" status. Basically, Medicare law provides that nonskilled custodial care may be covered by Medicare when neither the provider nor the patient had reason to know the services were not medically necessary.

The provider is allowed a certain percentage of wrong determinations before each admission decision is closely scrutinized by the Medicare intermediary. Up to that point, the provider is held harmless for wrong determinations and is not held liable for the costs. Therefore, it is important for the provider to maintain this favorable status.

In addition to making admission determinations, the SNF provider will also make decisions about continuing Medicare coverage. For example, a rehabilitation patient may be denied continued Medicare coverage after four weeks of physical therapy services. This decision is made by the SNF through its URC.

Technically, the URC is made up of at least two physicians, a registered nurse, and perhaps an administrator. It is the function of the URC to review the medical records and decide the appropriate level of care for each patient. However, in practice it is usually the nurse who makes the decision, at admission and upon continuing review, and then presents the assessments to the URC. The usual course is for the URC to approve the nurse's decisions after brief review sessions.

Although the patient's attending physician has the opportunity to meet with the URC and support the need for Medicare coverage, this does not happen often. In short, the usual URC function might be described as perfunctory with actual decisions being made by one or two nonphysician SNF staff persons.

Intermediary Decisions

The SNF must submit a billing to the Medicare intermediary to obtain an "official" denial of coverage. The initial notice provided by the provider is not a true denial of coverage. A bill must be submitted and the intermediary will then issue a denial notice to the beneficiary.

Accordingly, it is most important that the bill be submitted to the Medicare intermediary even when the SNF believes that services will not be covered. This procedure is referred to as no-payment billing.

All beneficiaries have the right to have bills submitted to Medicare, and SNF providers are obligated to submit the bills. A recent litigation settlement specifically provides that a SNF provider cannot bill the patient or a third party until a Medicare intermediary denial has been issued. This case also reinforces patients' rights to have no-payment bills submitted.

Although it is the intermediary that performs the first official assessment of a patient's level of care, in actuality the intermediary merely rubber-stamps the SNF provider denial. Therefore, if the provider issues a notice of noncoverage, the intermediary will also issue a notice of noncoverage. However, this practice is not reciprocated for approved admissions. An intermediary, through random audit, will review SNF admissions of covered Medicare stays.

The intermediary often reverses the SNF decision to grant Medicare coverage. However, the patient is protected by the limitation of liability provision because written notice of noncoverage was not given.

The reconsideration review is performed by the intermediary after the patient has been denied coverage. Many more medical records are available to document the services that have been provided. Now the intermediary can look back over the records to determine the level of care as opposed to looking ahead to determine what care a patient will require. This is true also for a coverage denial of continuing care after Medicare coverage was initially granted.

The medical records are reviewed by a staff person who was not involved in the initial decision. A recommendation is made to uphold or reverse the initial decision. The file is then reviewed by a physician or registered nurse acting as a medical consultant, who either agrees or disagrees with the recommendation. A written decision is then issued to the beneficiary.

In appeals for SNF services, the level of patient care is the deciding factor. The following basic requirements must be addressed when evaluating the availability of the SNF benefit:

- Only post-hospital admissions for skilled nursing or rehabilitation care are covered.

- Ordinarily, post-hospital transfer and skilled services must begin within 30 days after leaving the hospital.

- The skilled services must be provided daily on an inpatient basis.

- A maximum of 100 days per benefit period may be covered.

If all of these criteria are not satisfied, it is likely that you will not have good grounds for appeal. For example, if the patient receives skilled nursing care and custodial care but the skilled care is not daily, no grounds for appeal exist since the law specifies that the care must be needed on a daily basis. If the patient is not admitted within 30 days of discharge from the hospital (unless it is medically appropriate to delay the admission), the services will not be covered.

HOME HEALTH CARE SERVICES

A beneficiary who desires home health coverage must request Medicare-covered services from a home health agency certified by Medicare. Typically, the agency will evaluate the patient and determine whether coverage will be available for the needed care. If the agency believes coverage will be granted by the intermediary (the entity, usually an insurance company, acting as Medicare's agent), the agency will deliver the services and submit a claim for coverage to the intermediary. The claims are usually submitted at two-month intervals.

Whenever a home health agency submits a claim to the intermediary, it risks financial penalty. If the intermediary determines that the services involved should not be covered, it issues an initial determination denying the claim. The agency may not charge the patient for the cost of services delivered until the patient is informed, in writing, that Medicare coverage is denied. The agency is therefore forced to absorb the cost of the care involved.

The agency may avoid this penalty, however, if it has established a favorable "track record," demonstrating that it generally has been able to differentiate between coverable and noncoverable claims.

If fewer than two and a half percent of all claims submitted by an agency in a calendar quarter receive fiscal intermediary denials, the agency is entitled to a "presumption of no fault." This permits the intermediary to make payment for the care involved despite its noncoverable status.

The agency's percentage of claims denied is called the "denial rate." If the denial rate exceeds two and a half percent, the agency will be responsible for the cost of care in all cases where its claims submissions are denied by the intermediary.

Figure 6-9: Medicare Home Health Claims Submission and Appeals Process

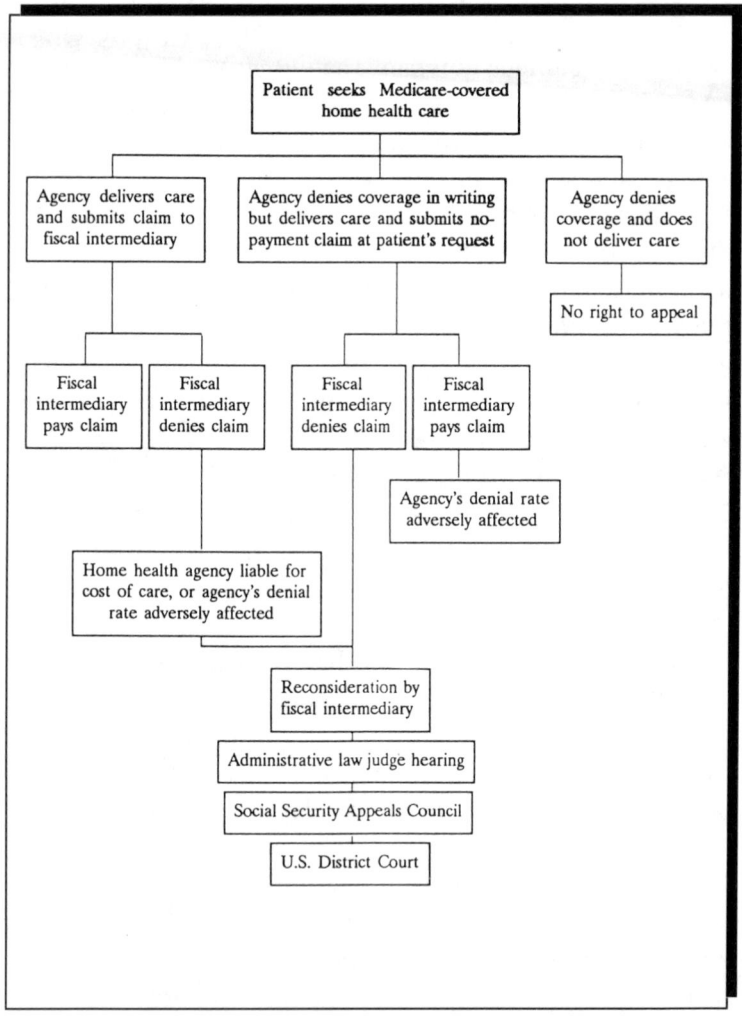

Figure 6-9 is reproduced with permission from the Legal Counsel for the Elderly, *Medicare Practice Manual* © 1990. The discussion following Figure 6-9 was adapted from the *Medicare Practice Manual* as well.

The calculation of the home health agency denial rate was liberalized somewhat in the Omnibus Budget Reconciliation Act of 1989 (OBRA '89); beginning on January 1, 1990, bills submitted by home health agencies will not be considered denied until the end of the 60-day period following the denial, or until the intermediary issues a reconsideration decision affirming the denial.

If the home health agency believes coverage will be denied by the intermediary, or when the agency is unsure whether coverage will be granted or denied, it will generally seek to escape any financial penalty by not submitting a claim. Although the beneficiary has a right to insist that a claim be submitted even where the home health agency believes coverage will be denied (called a no-payment claim), often the agency will discourage the patient from requiring such a submission because, under some circumstances, the agency may be penalized if the intermediary determines that a no-payment claim should have been deemed covered by the agency.

The claims submission and penalty process in the home health setting, and in other areas of Medicare, uses the waiver of liability system. The liability of the patient for the cost of care is waived until he or she is informed, in writing, that coverage is not available. In addition, the possibility that the agency will be forced to absorb the cost of care after an intermediary denial is waived if the agency did not exceed the denial rate in the previous quarter.

The net result of the waiver system is to force home health agencies to deny claims that should be granted coverage. In many cases, this system results in a complete lack of care as well as the loss of the right to appeal. When the agency is afraid to claim coverage from the intermediary, the agency usually will not deliver home health services unless the patient agrees to pay for them. If the patient cannot afford the care required, the care will not be provided even though Medicare coverage should have been granted, and could have been won on appeal had the care been delivered and a claim submitted (the intermediary will not make an initial determination on a claim until after the services have been rendered).

CHAPTER 7

THE APPEALS PROCESS
FOR PART B

Part B determinations, like Part A determinations, can be appealed. However, the processes are a little different so this chapter is devoted to explaining only Part B appeals.

Approximately two out of three Part B decisions are reversed at the first level of appeal. Therefore, it can be well worth your time to request an appeal.

Unfortunately, many beneficiaries believe they either cannot appeal a determination, or that it is too difficult to do. Also, many believe that the determination will not be changed anyway "so why bother?" However, the process is not really all that difficult.

GENERAL PRINCIPLES

Medicare law permits any party to a claim to file an appeal if he is dissatisfied with the determination made by the carrier. For assigned claims, your physician will file the appeal since you assigned your benefits to him. Although it may seem that your physician will be handling all appeals, there are two reasons you need the information provided in this chapter.

First, you can help your physician when he files an appeal for an assigned claim. You may be needed to provide information about your condition or treatment or other similar types of information. Second, physicians cannot appeal unassigned claims, which means you will need to file the appeal and follow through with it if you are dissatisfied with the carrier's determination.

The appeals process consists of three levels: the review, the fair hearing, and the administrative law judge (ALJ) hearing.

The claimant (the person requesting the appeal) can be either the beneficiary or the physician. For the physician to appeal, he must have accepted assignment on the claim in question. Or, if he did not accept assignment, the claim must have been denied on the basis that the services were not reasonable and necessary and the physician is being held liable for the charges.

An appeal must start at the lowest level (the review) and proceed "upward." This means that if the claimant is dissatisfied with the review determination, he moves to the next level, the fair hearing, and so on. The claimant cannot immediately request an ALJ hearing if he has not had a review and a fair hearing first.

Each level of appeal has two requirements: a time limit within which the appeal must be filed and a minimum dollar amount in question (also called the "amount in controversy"). Figure 7-1 outlines the time and amount in controversy limits for each level.

The time limit for filing an appeal can be extended if the claimant can show good cause why he did not file within the time limit. The same conditions that establish good cause for Part A appeals also apply to Part B appeals.

REVIEW

The first step in the appeals process is a simple one that involves very little work. You must request the review, in writing, within six months of the date of the initial determination. (The time limit is measured from the date on the EOMB.)

Figure 7-1: Time and Amount in Controversy Limits for Part B Appeals

Level	Time Limit	Minimum Amount in Controversy
Review	Within 6 months of the date of initial determination (as indicated on the EOMB or remittance advice)	None
Fair hearing	Within 6 months of the date of review determination	$100
ALJ hearing	Within 60 days of the date of the fair hearing decision	$500

Additional information can be submitted to help explain why the claimant feels the determination is in error. It is the claimant's responsibility to submit additional evidence to support the claim; don't expect the carrier to ask for it.

Carrier staff, who typically have prior claims processing experience, will then review the service(s) in question. They will look at the original claim information and any supporting evidence submitted. They also sometimes consult with consultants or medical personnel employed by the carrier. A decision is then rendered within 45 days of the request.

Many carriers now offer telephone reviews. Carriers will discuss the claim with you by phone and may be able to render a decision at that time. Check with your local carrier to see if this is available to you.

If the review decision results in payment of the claim, the carrier will forward a letter explaining its decision and include payment. If the physician requested the review, an informational copy is sent to the beneficiary. The physician may then collect the copayment and any unmet portion of the deductible from the patient.

How To Request and Prepare for a Review

The claimant for a review may be a beneficiary, an assignee (a physician who accepted assignment), or a designated representative. If the claimant wishes to be represented, he must file an Appointment of Representative form (see Figure 6-1 in Chapter Six).

All requests for review must be made in writing. Form HCFA-1964 (Figure 7-2) can be completed and used to request a review. These forms should be available from your carrier.

If you do not wish to use the form (it is not required), you can send a letter to the carrier. A sample letter for requesting a review is shown in Figure 7-3.

The claimant is responsible for submitting additional information. Some examples of information that would be helpful in supporting your request are:

- X-ray reports or films

- Test results

- Medical history of patient

- Documentation of severity of illness or acute onset

Figure 7-2: HCFA-1964—Request for Review of Part B Medicare Claim

---

DEPARTMENT OF HEALTH AND HUMAN SERVICES
HEALTH CARE FINANCING ADMINISTRATION

Form Approved
OMB No. 0938-0033

REQUEST FOR REVIEW OF PART B MEDICARE CLAIM
Medical Insurance Benefits – Social Security Act

NOTICE—Anyone who misrepresents or falsifies essential information requested by this form may upon conviction be subject to fine and imprisonment under Federal Law.

1	Carrier's Name and Address

2	Name of Patient

3	Health Insurance Claim Number

4 I do not agree with the determination you made on my claim as described on my Explanation of Medicare Benefits dated:

5 MY REASONS ARE: (Attach a copy of the Explanation of Medicare Benefits, or describe the service, date of service, and physician's name—NOTE —If the date on the Notice of Benefits mentioned in item 3 is more than six months ago, include your reason for not making this request earlier.)

6 Describe Illness or Injury:

7 ☐ I have additional evidence to submit. (Attach such evidence to this form.)

☐ I do not have additional evidence.

COMPLETE ALL OF THE INFORMATION REQUESTED. SIGN AND RETURN THE FIRST COPY AND ANY ATTACHMENTS TO THE CARRIER NAMED ABOVE. IF YOU NEED HELP, TAKE THIS AND YOUR NOTICE FROM THE CARRIER TO A SOCIAL SECURITY OFFICE, OR TO THE CARRIER. KEEP THE DUPLICATE COPY OF THIS FORM FOR YOUR RECORDS.

8

SIGNATURE OF **EITHER** THE CLAIMANT **OR** HIS REPRESENTATIVE

Representative	Claimant
Address	Address
City, State, and ZIP Code	City, State, and ZIP Code
Telephone Number	Date	Telephone Number	Date

Form HCFA-1964 (8-85)

Figure 7-3: Sample Letter to Request a Review

Department of Reviews
Carrier Name
Address
City, State, Zip

RE: Claim Number 999999999999
        Patient Name and HICN

Dear Sir or Madam:

I am requesting a review of the above claim. Specifically, please review the determination made on the following service(s): (Include description of service/procedure including code number, if appropriate).

I feel the determination is in error because (clearly state and fully explain reason).

I have enclosed a copy of the EOMB containing the determination for the claim in question and additional information to support my reasons for requesting this review.

If further information is needed, please feel free to contact me.

Thank you for your consideration.

Sincerely,

Name
Enclosures: Copy of EOMB

(List types of documentation included, e.g., consult report, operative notes)

- Consultation reports

- Billing forms

- Referrals

- Plan of treatment

- Nurse's notes

- Copies of communications between and among physicians, the beneficiary, hospital, laboratory, etc.

Carriers are instructed to assist claimants in obtaining information if they are having trouble getting it. If you have trouble obtaining the hospital's chart notes or the lab's test results, for example, tell the carrier. Not only will they be aware that you have additional information to submit, but they should help you obtain it.

This is important because, if the additional information is not received within 30 days of the review request, the review will be performed based on the information contained in the file. This means that the carrier will probably make the same determination that was made the first time the claim was processed because they have no new information to help them make a different determination.

Tips for a Successful Review

The key to a successful review is additional documentation. The carrier will almost be forced to make the same determination in a review as it did initially without good reason to do otherwise. Not only must you send additional information, but you should also take a little time to organize the information and think about the best way to present it to the reviewer.

For example, you should not send your entire medical chart and history; copy only those sections that apply to and justify the provision of the services in question. If your medical history is complicated and detailed, but you feel that it supports the services provided, *summarize* it on a separate piece of paper and include it with your request.

The goal is not to overwhelm the reviewer with the doctor's ability to keep good medical records; it is to provide justification for the service provided or the charge submitted. Don't be afraid to ask for your doctor's help in summarizing your medical information or providing other relevant information. Remember, he wants you to get paid as much as you want to get paid!

If you have a situation involving complicated services or procedures provided in a short period of time, ask your doctor to take a few minutes to write a letter. Ask that it be presented in lay terms, explaining your status, the reasons for each service/procedure, and what each service/procedure involved. Remember that the reviewer, although he may be experienced in analyzing claims and familiar with medical terminology, is not a physician or other medically trained person. Sending a letter that explains the situation simply and directly makes his job a little easier and helps him to make a decision in your favor.

Limit the scope of the review request. Don't send a letter that says "Please review this claim." Instead, specify the services that you want reviewed and provide specific documentation to support your belief that the initial determination was incorrect. Failure to be specific will result in a general review of the claim and could result in the carrier deciding that the initial determination for other services was incorrect.

Finally, don't be afraid to ask your doctor's office to help you. They can provide necessary documents, records, test results, etc., to help have the initial determination reversed. Also, the practice should have a vested interest in your obtaining payment for the services; if you don't get paid, it is much less likely that the doctor will get paid!

FAIR HEARING

The fair hearing is the second level of appeal. While the hearing is more formal than a review, it is not as formal as a traditional court hearing.

A claimant who is dissatisfied with the decision rendered in a review may request a hearing. The request must be submitted in writing, within six months of the date of the review decision. The hearing request should specify the type of hearing requested. There are three types of hearings: on-the-record, in-person, and telephone.

For a hearing, the amount in controversy must be $100 or more. To meet the $100 requirement, you may combine claims that have already been reviewed by the carrier. The amount in controversy minimum does not have to be reached with a single claim.

The claimant may be a beneficiary, an assignee (a physician who accepted assignment), or a designated representative. If the claimant wishes to be represented, he must file an Appointment of Representative (see Figure 6-1 in Chapter Six).

The hearing, which is conducted by a hearing officer (HO), affords the claimant the opportunity to discuss his dissatisfaction and present oral testimony. After the HO hears testimony and examines other relevant facts, he renders a decision within 30 days of the date of the hearing.

If the hearing results in payment to the claimant, the HO notifies the carrier. The carrier then has 15 days to "effectuate," or put into effect, the HO's decision and pay the claimant.

The Role of the Hearing Officer

It is important to understand the role of the hearing officer. Although he is employed by the carrier, he is directed to make an impartial decision based on the material presented. The HO has an incentive to make the "proper" decision because the HCFA Regional Office reviews the HO's decisions. Not only are the statistics tallied, but the Regional Office evaluates the quality of the hearing decisions as well. An HO can be a lawyer, but is typically selected by the carrier from its more qualified management staff.

Note that the HO can settle controversies involving only Part B benefits. He is not permitted to make decisions regarding any matter for which HCFA has sole responsibility, such as issues related to Part A benefits or the individual's entitlement to Part B benefits.

Some examples of the types of determinations that the HO has authority to make relate to:

- The reasonableness of a charge.

- Whether services were medically necessary.

- Whether items or services are covered.

- Whether the deductible has been met.

- Whether payment can be made under the limitation of liability provision.

- Whether a physician is without fault if the carrier held the physician liable for refunding an overpayment (for medically unnecessary services).

The HO must make a complete examination of the entire claim, including the reasonable charge calculation, the necessity of the services, coverage of the services, and any other relevant issues. This is done to "flush out" any errors that may have been overlooked in the initial processing or review determination. While this may seem like a drawback to filing for a hearing, it should encourage claimants to file more meaningful requests for hearings and to adequately prepare for the hearing.

Three Types of Fair Hearing

The claimant, not the HO, decides whether to request an in-person, telephone, or on-the-record hearing. Regardless of the type of fair hearing, the claimant should receive the same consideration; one type of hearing does not typically result in a more favorable decision than another. The types differ in the time and effort required of the claimant and the carrier, the way in which they are conducted, the method of presenting testimony, the speed with which they can be conducted, and the speed with which the decision can be rendered.

In-Person Hearing

An in-person hearing is one where the claimant meets with the HO. During an in-person hearing, the claimant and the carrier can present oral and written testimony, have witnesses testify, and challenge the testimony and evidence presented.

The advantages of an in-person hearing are the ability to challenge the evidence supplied and to present oral testimony. Presenting oral testimony can be a great advantage when there is some matter that needs to be clarified, because the HO can ask you questions and you can explain the details of your situation.

However, the in-person hearing can be time consuming and inconvenient and, in some cases, may be unnecessary if the claimant does not need or wish to present oral testimony. Also, some people may be uncomfortable in this type of situation.

Telephone Hearing

The telephone hearing differs from the in-person hearing only in that it is conducted over the phone (like a conference call) rather than in person. It is less time consuming (many telephone hearings only take about 15 minutes) and may feel less intimidating to the claimant.

On-The-Record Hearing

All requests for fair hearing are reviewed by the HO prior to the hearing. In effect, all cases may receive an on-the-record (OTR) decision. However, an OTR hearing can also be requested by the claimant if he does not wish to present oral testimony or does not wish to challenge the evidence provided by the carrier.

The only difference between an OTR hearing and the other two types of hearings is that no oral testimony is presented. The HO simply evaluates the claim based on the information contained in the file and then renders a decision.

An OTR hearing very closely resembles a review, except that the decision is made by an HO rather than a claims reviewer. For those who are uncomfortable with presenting oral testimony or who do not feel oral testimony is warranted, the OTR hearing can result in a faster decision with less work for the claimant.

How To Request a Fair Hearing

A fair hearing must be requested within six months of the review determination. Under no circumstances can a hearing be requested if a review has not already been performed.

The request must be received in writing and should specify the type of hearing requested. You can use HCFA Form-1965 (Figure 7-4) to request a fair hearing, although it is not required. The form should be available from your carrier.

If you do not wish to use the form, you can send a letter to the carrier. A sample letter for requesting a fair hearing is provided in Figure 7-5.

As with reviews, the claimant is responsible for submitting additional information. If you do not submit the information with your request for hearing, you have ten days to forward it to the HO. Failure to forward the information will result in the HO rendering a decision based on the information in the file.

Figure 7-4: Form HCFA-1965—Request for Fair Hearing, Part B
Medicare Claim

DEPARTMENT OF HEALTH AND HUMAN SERVICES
HEALTH CARE FINANCING ADMINISTRATION

Form Approved
OMB No. 0836-0034

REQUEST FOR HEARING – PART B MEDICARE CLAIM
Medical Insurance Benefits – Social Security Act

NOTICE—Anyone who misrepresents or falsifies essential information requested by this form may upon conviction
be subject to fine and imprisonment under Federal Law.

Carrier's Name and Address	**1** Name of Patient
	2 Health Insurance Claim Number

3 I disagree with the review determination on my claim, and request a hearing before a hearing officer of the
insurance carrier named above.

MY REASONS ARE: *(Attach a copy of the Review Notice. NOTE —If the review decision was made
more than 6 months ago, include your reason for not making this request earlier.)*

_____

_____

_____

_____

4 Check one of the Following:

☐ I have additional evidence to submit.
*(Attach such evidence to this form
or forward it to the carrier within 10 days.)*

☐ I do not have additional evidence.

Check Only One of the Statements Below:

☐ I wish to appear in person before the
Hearing Officer.

☐ I do not wish to appear and hereby
request a decision on the evidence
before the Hearing Officer.

5 EITHER THE CLAIMANT OR REPRESENTATIVE SHOULD SIGN IN THE APPROPRIATE SPACE BELOW:

Signature or Name of Claimant's Representative	Claimant's Signature
➔	➔
Address	Address
City, State, and ZIP Code	City, State, and ZIP Code
Telephone Number	Date	Telephone Number	Date

(Claimant should not write below this line)

ACKNOWLEDGMENT OF REQUEST FOR HEARING

Your request for a hearing was received on _____ . You will be notified of the time and
place of the hearing at least 10 days before the date of the hearing.

Signed	Date

Form HCFA-1965 (8-79)

Figure 7-5: Sample Letter to Request a Fair Hearing

Hearing Officer
Department of Hearings
Carrier Name
Address
City, State, Zip

RE: Claim Number(s) 999999999999
     Patient Name(s) and HICN(s)

Dear Sir or Madam:

I am requesting a fair hearing of the above claim(s) as I am dissatisfied with the review determination. I would like to have (an in-person, a telephone, an on-the-record) hearing. In the hearing, please review the determination made on the following service(s): (include description of service/procedure including code number, if appropriate).

I feel the determination is in error because (clearly state and fully explain reason).

I have enclosed (indicate and describe type(s) of additional supporting information) to support my reasons for requesting this hearing.

If further information is needed, please feel free to contact me. Thank you for your consideration.

Sincerely,

Name
Encl.:   Copy of EOMB
         Copy of Review Determination
(List types of documentation included, e.g., consult report, operative notes, summary of patient's condition.)

The carrier must acknowledge your request for a fair hearing within ten days of receipt of your request. Your file is then forwarded to the HO assigned to the hearing.

The HO will contact you, in writing, to inform you about the hearing process and to schedule a date for an in-person or telephone hearing, if one was requested. You should receive notification about the time and place for the hearing at least 14 days before the date of the hearing. If an OTR hearing was requested, the HO will proceed with the decision upon receipt of the file.

The Hearing Officer's Preparation

The carrier forwards all pertinent documents related to the claim to the HO. The carrier can also submit additional information to justify the initial determination. The regulations instruct the HO to prepare for the hearing by examining the evidence in the file, including any material submitted with the hearing request.

According to the regulations, after the HO verifies the claimant's eligibility for the hearing, the completeness of the evidence, and the issues to be determined, he then examines sections of the law, regulations, rulings, policy statements, general instructions, and other formal guides as they apply to the issues to be determined in the hearing. After reviewing the evidence, the HO notifies the parties to the hearing, including the beneficiary if the claimant is a physician, and any other appointed representative.

At this point, the HO has many choices regarding how to proceed. He can:

- Dismiss the request. A request for hearing can be dismissed for several reasons:

- The amount in controversy limit is not satisfied.

- The claim(s) are not at the proper level of appeal.

- The claimant is not a proper party to the hearing.

- The claimant died and there is no information to show that any other party may be prejudiced by the last (review) determination.

- The claimant requests an in-person hearing but does not appear and does not show good and sufficient cause within ten days for not appearing or for not notifying the HO that he could not appear.

- The claimant requests a telephone hearing but fails to participate at the scheduled time and does not show good and sufficient cause for not having participated or for not having notified the HO that he could not participate.

• Remand the claim to the carrier for payment and dismissal. If the carrier determines that the claim can be paid after forwarding the file to the HO, the carrier can request dismissal of the request and pay the claim.

• Accept a withdrawal at the request of the claimant or representative. The claimant can withdraw his request at any time before the mailing of the hearing decision. The claimant must request the withdrawal in writing.

- Transfer the request to another carrier's HO if an out-of-area hearing has been requested. This occurs if the claimant is not located in the HO's geographic area.

- Transfer the request to the Regional Office if the issues are outside the HO's authority to determine. For example, if the issue is the beneficiary's eligibility for Part B benefits, the HO does not have the authority to make this determination and must forward the file to the Regional Office.

- Conduct the hearing. In this case, the HO continues with the hearing process.

How You Should Prepare

You will first need to decide what type of fair hearing you prefer. The discussion above outlined some of the advantages and disadvantages of each type. To make your decision, consider the time it may take to carry out each type and whether or not you will feel comfortable presenting oral testimony.

If presenting oral testimony does not disturb you and you feel that witnesses, such as your physician or practitioner, would be helpful to your case, an in-person hearing is warranted. If you feel that an oral explanation (in addition to the written documentation you provide) to the HO would adequately defend your position, you may want to consider the telephone hearing. Many find the telephone hearing beneficial because it takes less time and seems less intimidating than the more formal in-person hearing.

If you believe that the documentation you provided for the review, plus some additional written information, will convince the HO in your favor, then you may want to consider the on-the-record hearing.

In any case, the key is to prepare. Don't expect that the HO will grant a reversal based on your feeling that the previous decision was in error. You have to *prove* to him that the determination should be reversed.

In addition to the documentation you prepared for the review, you should provide additional written information, such as an explanation of the circumstances surrounding your claim, or additional reasons you feel the review decision was not correct. Remember, the information you provided for the review did not achieve the result you wanted and, therefore, must not have been adequate to support your position. So, prepare more material.

Also, it will be helpful to do some research on the regulations, rules, and laws that apply to your claim. You need to understand how the regulations affect the issues at your hearing so that you will be able to adequately defend your position. The fact that you are aware of this information should help, because the HO will see that you are prepared and well-informed.

Under the regulations for fair hearings, the claimant has the right to review all material contained in the HO's file prior to the hearing. If the HO does not send this information to you when you schedule a time for your hearing, be sure to request it. In some cases, the hearing could be scheduled as soon as 30 days after receipt of your request, which may not provide a great deal of time to prepare.

Once you receive the file, review it carefully. It will contain the carrier's reasons for denying your claim initially and at the review. Use this information to your advantage by preparing a logical, well-organized argument to refute the carrier's position.

You should also have a good understanding of the fair hearing procedures, rules of questioning, and proper conduct at the hearing. If you walk into your hearing with an argumentative attitude and have to keep interrupting to ask questions because you do not know what's going on, the HO will be less inclined to help you. Anticipating the needs of the HO, understanding how the hearing will proceed, and having your arguments and support documentation organized will go a long way in helping you to win a reversal.

The Fair Hearing Procedure

Before any telephone or in-person hearings are held, the HO makes an on-the-record decision. An OTR decision is rendered regardless of the type of hearing requested, unless the HO feels that he cannot make a fair decision without hearing oral testimony.

If the claimant requested an in-person or telephone hearing, the HO includes the date and time of the hearing with his decision letter. A postcard is also included, which the claimant uses to either confirm the date and time of the in-person or telephone hearing or to accept the decision rendered in the OTR determination. Failure to respond to the HO regarding your choice could cause the OTR decision to become final.

If you do not agree with the OTR decision and you still want an in-person or telephone hearing, return the postcard affirming that you will be present at the hearing. If the OTR decision is acceptable to you, return the postcard indicating that you accept the OTR decision and do not require an in-person or telephone hearing.

Claimants can waive their right to appear. If the parties waive their right to an in-person or telephone hearing, the

HO makes an on-the-record decision. A request for a telephone hearing or an on-the-record decision is a waiver of the right to an in-person hearing.

The parties can withdraw the waiver at any time *prior* to the issuance of the hearing decision. This means a claimant who elects an in-person or telephone hearing but then chooses not to appear (accepts the OTR decision initially rendered by the HO) will not be allowed to choose the in-person or telephone hearing later. A decision has been rendered.

At no time can the HO require a certain type of hearing. He may suggest a telephone hearing in cases of adverse weather conditions or if the claimant must travel a great distance, but he cannot require you to have a telephone or other type of hearing. Only if the claimant fails to confirm that he will attend the in-person or telephone hearing by failure to return the postcard (and fails to respond after the HO further attempts to contact him regarding his choice) can the claimant be forced to accept the OTR hearing.

Rules of the Fair Hearing

There are some significant differences between a Medicare fair hearing and a traditional court hearing. The procedure applies to both telephone and in-person hearings.

First, the hearing is non-adversarial in nature. Neither the carrier nor HCFA opposes the claimant; they are interested in a proper decision. Therefore, formal objections and other accepted court procedural tactics are not appropriate.

Second, rules of evidence and proof are less restrictive and their emphasis is different from those used in court.

Third, the HO's role is that of a trier of the facts and he considers as evidence any testimony or documentation that enables him to make a correct decision. During hearings, the HO questions participants to develop evidence and establish facts.

Finally, new evidence may be presented throughout the hearing, witnesses may be asked to testify again, parties need not make a final statement, and a party always has the right of rebuttal after evidence adverse to his case has been presented. When new evidence is presented at the hearing, parties have the opportunity to read it and offer comments.

These procedures differ from a traditional court hearing in that they are less formal and restrictive. Everyone gets a chance to talk, to defend his case, and to continue to present evidence even though it may not have been sent to the HO prior to the hearing.

Do not assume this means you can wait to present all your evidence at the hearing. Preparation and advance information to the HO will impress the HO that you are taking the proceeding seriously and have taken the time to prepare.

Rights of the Parties

The regulations guarantee certain rights to all parties to a fair hearing. All claimants have the right to:

* Present oral arguments and/or written statements as testimony.

* Be represented by an attorney or other qualified individual (representation by counsel is optional, not required).

- Bring witnesses to testify on their behalf.

- Bring and present all evidence in their possession, including pertinent records, documents, or other information affecting the issues.

- Question witnesses and other parties.

- Examine the evidence prior to the hearing.

- Register objections to the inclusion of any document in the record.

What Happens During the Hearing

As in a traditional court hearing, the fair hearing proceeding is recorded, either by a stenographer or tape recording. Typically, both the stenographer and the tape recording are used for both the telephone and the in-person hearing. This ensures that all information shared and discussed is captured. The HO will inform the parties if the discussion is being taped. The transcript of the hearing is available to the parties after the close of the hearing.

After introducing the parties to the hearing and recording their names, etc., in the record, the HO will begin the proceeding with an opening statement, which contains a summary of the purpose of the hearing, the issues involved, the rights of the parties, a statement regarding penalties for presenting false information or statements, and some procedural information.

A party may disagree with the HO's summary; if warranted, the HO may modify it. The HO has no authority to administer oaths. However, stiff penalties exist for those who present false or misleading information.

The hearing then begins. Usually, the HO does the majority of the questioning, striving to pinpoint the issues and gather the relevant evidence. Generally, the claimant is allowed to render testimony first.

After the hearing begins, certain circumstances may warrant a continuance:

- Certain testimony or a document submitted at the hearing takes the claimant or other party by surprise, is adverse to his interests, and presents evidence that he could not reasonably have anticipated and is not prepared to address.

- The HO enlarges the issues and either the claimant or another party or the HO needs to obtain additional evidence.

- New evidence is submitted during a telephone hearing, requiring time for all parties to examine and evaluate it and respond, if appropriate.

It is advisable for you to request a continuance only when you are not prepared to respond to the material presented.

If no continuance is requested and all testimony is heard, the HO closes the hearing and the HO writes a decision letter. If, after the close of the hearing, new evidence is presented that adversely affects the claimant, the HO must reopen the hearing to give the claimant an opportunity to respond. This does not mean that everyone has to meet again, only that the claimant has the opportunity to write a response to the new evidence.

The decision must be rendered within 30 days of the hearing. The decision letter should include a statement of the service(s) and issue(s) in question; a summary of the pertinent facts; the decision; a brief explanation of the basis for the decision, including proper reference to law, regulations, and policy applicable to the case; and a statement providing information about further appeal rights.

If a hearing involved assigned claims for more than one beneficiary, the HO forwards a copy of the decision to the physician and to each beneficiary as it pertains to each beneficiary's claim.

Tips for a Successful Fair Hearing

Preparation, preparation, preparation! The importance of adequately preparing for a fair hearing cannot be stressed enough. Preparation at this level involves not just making photocopies of the medical record, chart notes, or other relevant medical information, but also considering the *reasons* the carrier denied the claim initially and at the review. Take time to analyze your case from all angles and then assemble documentation that refutes the carrier's position.

Presentation—how you present your evidence and how you present yourself—is another important aspect of a successful hearing. Support documentation should be easy to read, easy to understand, and should clearly delineate the facts as you see them. Don't send a copy that is too dark, too light, or blurry. Don't send "scribbles" that are supposed to suffice for chart notes. If something is hard to read, re-type it. If your copier makes poor photocopies, go out and pay to make clear copies. Documentation that is sloppy may make the HO think your case is sloppy, too.

If you choose an in-person hearing, arrive on time (or early), have all your notes and documentation with you, and dress nicely. A claimant who shows up late or without all the necessary information will appear to the HO to have little respect for the proceeding or for the other parties involved. Again, a sloppy personal appearance may indicate a sloppy case.

When talking with the HO, be professional, explain your case articulately, and remain calm and logical. It will not pay to get emotional, lose your temper, or be insulting to the HO. A claimant who understands the issues and who has invested time in preparing his defense will make a better impression on the HO. Moreover, a good presentation should help you feel calmer and stay more focused on the issue at hand.

Finally, elicit the support of a witness if necessary. If the claim is for a complicated set of procedures or services, or the circumstances surrounding your medical condition are complicated, a witness such as your physician or another physician, can add credibility to your claim.

A last word about hearings—try not to let the process intimidate you. It is not terribly complicated nor is it tremendously difficult to prepare for and to execute. Don't be afraid to ask the HO for help; you may be surprised at how much help he can be. Remember, a hearing is a right available to you. You should feel confident using it when the situation calls for it.

ADMINISTRATIVE LAW JUDGE HEARING

The third level of appeal, the administrative law judge (ALJ) hearing, is actually not much different in concept from the fair hearing, except that the HO is replaced by an administrative law judge. An ALJ is a hearing official assigned to the Office of Hearings and Appeals of the Social Security Administration, while an HO is employed by a carrier.

The ALJ has a role and responsibilities similar to those of the HO in terms of the conduct of the hearing. Depending upon the circumstances, the procedural aspects of an ALJ hearing may differ from judge to judge.

How To Request an ALJ Hearing

If you are dissatisfied with the fair hearing decision, you may request an ALJ hearing. You must request it within 60 days of the date you receive the fair hearing decision and the amount in controversy must be at least $500.

To meet the $500 requirement, you may combine claims for the ALJ hearing if you have received a hearing officer's decision on all the claims, and you want an ALJ hearing on them, and the requests for an ALJ hearing are filed on time for each claim in the request. The amount in controversy minimum does not have to be reached with a single claim.

Also, to meet the $500 requirement, two or more people may combine claims if they were denied or had payment reduced for the same reasons.

To request an ALJ hearing, you must send a written request to the HO who heard your case; he will then forward it within ten working days to the ALJ. You can use the form shown in Figure 7-3 or use a letter of request similar to the one shown in Figure 7-6.

After receipt of your request, the HO will review the file again to determine whether a reversal is possible. If he determines that it is, the request for an ALJ hearing will be dismissed and you will be notified of the reversal. If the HO does not determine that a reversal is warranted, he will forward the case file to an ALJ at the Office of Hearings and Appeals.

Figure 7-6: Sample Letter to Request an ALJ Hearing

Hearing Officer/Administrative Law Judge
Department of Hearings
Carrier Name
Address
City, State, Zip

RE: Claim Number(s) 999999999999
       Patient Name and HICN

Dear Sir or Madam:

I am requesting an ALJ hearing of the above claim(s) as I am dissatisfied with the fair hearing determination. In the hearing, please review the determination made on the following service(s): (include a description of service/procedure including code number, if appropriate).

I feel the determination is in error because (clearly state and fully explain reason).

I have enclosed (indicate and describe type(s) of additional supporting information) to support my reasons for requesting this hearing. If further information is needed, please feel free to contact me.

Thank you for your consideration.

Sincerely,

Name
Encl.:   Copy of EOMB
          Copy of Review Determination
          Copy of Fair Hearing Determination
(List types of documentation included, e.g., consult report, operative notes, summary of patient's condition.)

In fiscal year 1993, HCFA reported that only 362,626 requests were received at the ALJ level. While statistics regarding reversals at this level are unavailable (due to the method of reporting), we can assume, based on reversal rates at the other two levels, that approximately one out of two cases received reversals.

How To Prepare for an ALJ Hearing

The same rules of preparation that applied to reviews and fair hearings apply to ALJ hearings. The regulations are very specific in outlining the information that the HO is required to send to the ALJ. The case file should include:

- The Medicare claim form with all relevant attachments or facsimile (printout) of an electronically generated claim.

- A copy of the EOMB or facsimile showing the original payment date.

- Documentation relating to any reopenings.

- The Request for Review form (HCFA-1964) or request letter with all attachments.

- Any other pertinent documents.

- Opinions of medical consultants or other experts who provided advice.

- A copy of the carrier's review determination.

- The Request for Fair Hearing form (HCFA-1965) or request letter with all attachments.

- An Appointment of Representative form (HCFA-1696-U4) or other authorization forms (if applicable).

- Medical information considered by the carrier's reviewer or HO, including treatment notes or summaries, physician's certification of medical necessity, doctor's orders or progress notes.

- Copies of law and regulations not otherwise referenced in the carrier's decision on which the carrier relied.

- Copies of carrier manual issuances and carrier policy statements on which the carrier relied.

- A copy of the dated fair hearing decision.

- If the fair hearing was taped, a copy of the tape; if a written transcript was prepared, a copy of the transcript.

- Original request for ALJ hearing. This must be signed by the claimant.

- New evidence provided with the ALJ request.

- An explanation or key to interpreting carrier-generated computer printouts.

- Documentation where there is a physician indemnification (under Section 1842(1)(1)(a)) issue, including documentation of whether the physician supplied adequate advance notice and a copy of the notice, if applicable.

As you can see by this list, the ALJ is provided with a great deal of information. You can use this list to help you prepare for the hearing since it points out the types of information the ALJ will be reviewing.

After the ALJ receives your request and the case file, he will contact you to schedule a time and date for the hearing. If at this time the ALJ does not provide you with details concerning the hearing, it is advisable that you ask him any questions you may have, since procedures vary from judge to judge. Also, when scheduling a date for your hearing, be sure to allow adequate time to prepare your case.

AFTER THE APPEALS PROCESS IS EXHAUSTED

After the appeals process is exhausted, a claimant has two more options: (1) appeal to the Appeals Council in Washington D.C., which is an administrative council within the Social Security Administration, or (2) take the case to the civil court system. It is not known how many claimants actually exercise these two options. HCFA does not keep statistics about these activities because they happen so rarely.

However, it is possible to appeal to the Appeals Council if you are unhappy with the ALJ's decision. The Appeals Council typically only hears cases where the claimant does not have enough in controversy to pursue the case in civil court.

If you wish to take your case to the courts, you need to have at least $1000 in controversy. Further information about this type of action should be obtained through a discussion with your attorney.

CHAPTER 8

FRAUD AND ABUSE

In the last few years, the terms "fraud" and "abuse" have been heard more and more frequently. Television news programs report on abuses and outright rip-offs of many federal programs, including Medicare.

The Office of the Inspector General (the independent office of the Department of Health and Human Services responsible for investigating fraud and abuse) has made a strong effort to educate the public about fraud and abuse and encourage beneficiaries and others to report instances of suspected fraud or abuse to the local Medicare carrier or intermediary.

While all this attention has helped the government slow these activities, it has also created a "bandwagon" on which everyone wants to jump. We are now very suspicious of our physicians, laboratories, and other providers of health care services, thinking they are all out to make a buck and don't care about treating the patient. This is unfortunate *and* untrue.

Statistics indicate that only about three percent of all suspected fraud and abuse reports have any actual merit as possible fraudulent or abusive acts. The remaining 97 percent are simply misunderstandings. Since beneficiaries account for a large percentage of reports, this chapter is provided to help educate you about the types of actions that can be considered fraud or abuse. You will be a better "watchdog" of the system, without causing the system undue work.

Please note that the term "provider" is used in this chapter to include all providers of health care, including physicians and other practitioners, suppliers, and hospitals.

FRAUD AND ABUSE DEFINED

Fraud

Fraud is defined as "*intentional* deception or misrepresentation that the individual makes, *knowing* it to be false, and that could result in some *unauthorized benefit* to them" (Section 14002.4B). Prior to April 1993, when this definition was clarified, a person could be considered to have committed fraud if he knew, or *should have known*, that the claim was false. The revised definition is not so "wishy-washy"; it is now clear that intent is a necessary element for conviction.

Some examples of fraudulent activities as they are defined in the regulations are:

- Billing for services or supplies that were not provided. This includes billing Medicare for services that were not actually furnished because the patient failed to keep his appointment (no-shows).

- Misrepresenting the diagnosis for the patient to justify the services or equipment furnished.

- Altering claim forms to obtain a higher reimbursement amount.

- Deliberately applying for duplicate reimbursement, for example, billing both Medicare and the beneficiary for the same service or billing both Medicare and another insurer in an attempt to get paid twice.

- Soliciting, offering, or receiving a kickback, bribe, or rebate, for example, paying for a referral of patients in exchange for the ordering of diagnostic tests and other services or medical equipment. (Routine waiver of coinsurance and/or the deductible falls into this classification.)

- Unbundled or exploded charges, for example, the billing of a multichannel set of lab tests to appear as if the individual tests had been performed.

- Completing Certificates of Medical Necessity (CMNs) for patients not personally and professionally known by the provider.

- Misrepresenting the services rendered (use of procedure codes not appropriate for the item or service actually furnished), amounts charged for services rendered, identity of the person receiving the services, dates of services, etc.

- Billing for noncovered services as covered services, for example, billing routine foot care as a more involved form of foot care to obtain reimbursement.

- Claims involving collusion between a physician and a beneficiary, or between a supplier and a physician, resulting in higher costs or charges to the Medicare program.

- Use of another person's Medicare card to obtain medical care.

- Alteration of claims history records to generate fraudulent payments.

- False provider disclosures of ownership in a clinical laboratory.

- Split billing schemes, for example, billing procedures over a period of days when all treatment occurred during one visit.

- Repeated violations of the participation agreement, assignment agreement, or the limiting charge provisions.

- Use of the adjustment process to generate fraudulent payments.

- Collusion between a provider and a carrier employee where the claim is assigned. (If the provider deliberately overbilled for services, adjustments could be generated with little awareness on the part of the beneficiary.)

- A carrier employee acting on his own behalf where the claim is unassigned. (Through manipulation of beneficiary address or the claims history record, a carrier employee could generate adjustment payments against many beneficiary records and cause payments to be mailed to an address known only to him).

- Billings based on "gang visits," for example, a physician visits a nursing home and bills for 20 nursing home visits without rendering any specific service to or on behalf of individual patients.

While not specifically itemized, altering your doctor's prescription can also be considered fraud. For example, changing a prescription for a wheelchair to one for a motorized wheelchair with extra padding can be considered fraud under the "altering claim forms" category.

Because an activity does not appear on this list does not mean that it could not be considered fraud. Any intentional attempt to defraud the Medicare program, or to provide care that is not consistent with professionally accepted standards, can expose a provider to liability.

Abuse

Abuse is defined as incidents or practices of providers, physicians, or suppliers that are inconsistent with accepted sound medical practices. Abuse may directly or indirectly result in unnecessary costs to the program, improper reimbursement, or payment for services that fail to meet professionally recognized standards of care or that are medically unnecessary.

Abuse involves payment for items or services when there is no legal entitlement to that payment and the provider has not knowingly and intentionally misrepresented facts to obtain payment. Activities that could be considered abuse are:

- Excessive charges for services or supplies.

- Claims for services not medically necessary, or not medically necessary to the extent furnished (e.g., a battery of diagnostic tests is given where, based on the diagnosis, only a few are needed).

- Physician exceeds limiting charge.

- Physician bills Medicare at a higher and different fee schedule rate than for non-Medicare patients. (HMOs and other special arrangements are not applicable for this provision.)

- Improper billing practices, including submittal of bills to Medicare instead of third-party payers that are primary insurers for Medicare beneficiaries.

- Violations of the Medicare participation agreement.

Some activities, such as breaches of the assignment agreement and violations of the participation agreement, appear as examples of both abuse and fraud. While these activities might sometimes be excused due to "ignorance," repeated violations after a warning could move from the abuse list to the fraud category.

It is important to realize that the Medicare program cannot investigate a physician or other provider for poor quality of care. If you feel that your physician is not providing you with adequate care, discuss it with him. If you are still not satisfied, report it to the state medical society. From Medicare's point of view, issues of abuse focus on inappropriate payment, not inappropriate care.

Forgery

Since federal funds are involved, all cases of alleged forgery are investigated to determine whether in fact the beneficiary or provider did receive the Medicare funds. The following situations indicate possible forgery:

- A beneficiary or provider states that he did not receive the Medicare check but the carrier shows that it was cashed.

- The endorsement on the back of the check does not match the name on the front.

- The payee claims that the signature on the check is not his.

IDENTIFYING FRAUD AND ABUSE ACTIVITIES

Your participation in and understanding of your own health care provides you with many benefits, including your good or improved health. Another benefit, however trivial compared to your health, is your contribution to the economics of health care. This includes the detection, investigation, and prosecution of those individuals or entities who take advantage of the system.

Fraud and abuse costs all of us money. So, to make your contribution as an informed patient and consumer of health care, you need to understand how to identify situations that could truly be considered fraud or abuse and then report them to the correct entity.

Know the Rules

The first step is familiarize yourself with activities which are considered fraudulent and abusive. The lists provided above are good places to start. Pamphlets and other information disseminated by the Office of the Inspector General (OIG) about specific fraudulent activities are also good references. Finally, your local Social Security office is another source to help you determine whether a situation should be considered fraud or abuse and reported.

Next you must become familiar with how the system works. Physicians and other providers must follow many rules and regulations when billing Medicare. If you are not at least familiar with the language and the process, you could very easily make an assumption that fraud has taken place. The more you understand, the better you will be able to identify when activities are possibly fraudulent or abusive.

The third thing you need to know is when to call your doctor's office to discuss something you don't understand on your bill and when to notify the carrier that a possible fraud situation exists. In many cases, your doctor is the best source of information to help you understand why something was billed the way it was and whether the charges are legitimate.

In addition, there are many beneficiary advocacy programs throughout the United States that should be able to help you if you have a question. All states have an insurance department and some type of agency on aging. A list of these agencies is provided in Appendix D.

Common Situations That May Not Be Fraud

As stated earlier in this chapter, only about two to three percent of complaints received from beneficiaries are legitimate. In the vast majority of cases, the complaint stems from the beneficiary's misunderstanding of how services are billed. To help prevent you from making an erroneous report, this section provides some of the most common complaints received by carriers and the explanations for each.

Complaint: *"I did not see this doctor."*

This is probably one of the most common complaints received. In many cases, the patient did not actually see the doctor, but the services are still legitimate. Instances where this could be true but where no fraud has occurred include:

- You have X-rays taken. An X-ray technician performs the X-rays; no physician is present. When you see that a physician (a radiologist) has been paid, you wonder why since he was not present. This practice is common. Technicians are not qualified to read the results (the film) of your X-rays; radiologists read X-rays and provide reports on their findings. They are allowed to bill for this service, even though they did not actually see you face to face.

- Following the X-ray example above, you see two charges for X-rays: one from a radiologist and one from the hospital. Is this fraud? Not likely.

  Medicare requires that the person or entity that performs a service bill only for that service. Since not many physicians maintain X-ray equipment in their office, but refer the work to a radiology group or the hospital, radiological services are billed in two parts. One part is for the technical component, which includes costs for taking the X-ray, such as use of the equipment, the film, etc. The other part is for the professional component, which includes the services only the doctor can provide such as interpreting the X-ray and reporting on the findings.

If you see two charges for an X-ray, it is likely that you are seeing the charges for each component of the service.

- You have surgery in a hospital and general anesthesia is used. For this service, there will be three bills: one from the hospital for use of the operating suite; one from the doctor for the actual surgical procedure; and one from the anesthesiologist for administering the anesthesia.

  Many patients do not realize that the anesthesiologist will bill separately from the hospital. They think this charge will be included in the hospital bill. It is not. As long as you had surgery and had anesthesia for the surgery, a bill from the anesthesiologist is appropriate (even though you may not remember this doctor).

- You fall down and break your hip, which requires you to have a total hip replacement. Your regular doctor recommends a surgeon who performs the surgery. Upon receiving the EOMB, you notice that two surgeons were paid for the surgery, but you do not know who the other doctor is.

In this case, if you can determine that the second surgeon was paid 16 percent of the amount the primary surgeon was paid, you can safely assume that surgeon was the assistant. Assistant surgeons are commonly used to help the primary surgeon. If you are still not convinced, contact the primary surgeon to verify that he did indeed use the doctor listed as his assistant during the surgery.

• You go to the hospital (as an outpatient) to have a biopsy performed on your breast. For this service, there will be three bills: one from the hospital for use of the operating suite; one from the doctor for the procedure; and one from the pathologist who looks at the tissue sample and determines whether it is malignant or benign.

Again, many patients do not realize that their doctor is not truly qualified to make this determination so the tissue sample must be analyzed by a doctor trained in this type of work. So, even though you do not actually see this doctor, his charge is legitimate.

Because of the way billing is handled, the above examples illustrate very common complaints received by carriers that turn out to be legitimate charges. However, should you notice that Medicare has paid for an X-ray or an X-ray interpretation and you have not had any X-rays, or if you see that Medicare has paid for anesthesia or interpretation of a lab sample and you have not recently been anesthetized nor had any lab work (e.g., blood or urine analyzed), it is possible that inappropriate billing is occurring. Report these incidents to your carrier.

Complaint: *"I did not receive this service or this many of a particular service."*

Many times it will appear that you have been charged for a service you did not receive or that you have been charged more than once for a particular service. As explained above in the discussion of professional and technical components of X-rays, this may be explained by the method used to bill radiological services. Also, if you have an X-ray performed where a dye is injected into your system, there will be a separate charge for the injection of the dye; this is not duplicate billing or fraud.

Another example is the repair of wounds or removal of some types of skin growths. Because of the wording in the coding manual, physicians must report repairs of wounds and growth removals separately when they are done on different parts of the body. Do not assume that the doctor has billed twice for a service as this may be the explanation.

Complaint: *"My carrier just sent me a letter asking for information about services I received from my doctor. Does this mean the doctor is being investigated for fraud?"*

Not usually. Carriers are required to perform routine "audits" of physicians and it is possible that your physician was selected. The carrier is simply verifying that the services were provided as reported.

MEDICARE'S POLICE FORCE

The Roles of the Different Agencies

Everyone from the Health Care Financing Administration (HCFA) to the beneficiary is considered part of the Medicare "police force." According to the regulations:

The Medicare program pays for health care items and services for millions of beneficiaries and provides payment to tens of thousands of providers and suppliers [physicians, practitioners] of services. Within a program of such complexity and magnitude, the opportunities for fraud, abuse, and waste are considerable. The quality control effort to detect and eliminate fraud, abuse, and waste is necessarily a cooperative effort involving the beneficiaries, contractors [carriers and intermediaries], PROs, state Medicaid agencies, and Federal agencies such as HCFA and the Office of the Inspector General (OIG), Department of Health and Human Services (DHHS).

Medicare enlists all agencies and people that have contact with the program. This section looks at the agencies involved in overseeing Medicare, and describes their roles, responsibilities, and authority in detecting and pursuing cases.

The Health Care Financing Administration

HCFA is the administrator of the Medicare program. While HCFA is not actively involved in investigations, it does provide guidelines (the regulations) that the carriers and intermediaries (and other agencies and organizations HCFA oversees) use to detect and pursue cases of fraud and abuse.

HCFA also maintains Regional Offices that conduct program reviews designed to prevent improper expenditures of Medicare funds and ensure that program payments are made only in the proper amounts. Regional Offices are rarely involved in the investigation process.

The Office of the Inspector General (OIG)

The OIG is an independent office of Department of Health and Human Services (DHHS). Under the Social Security Act, it has responsibility for protecting the integrity of departmental programs as well as the health and welfare of beneficiaries served by those programs.

Through a comprehensive program of audits, inspections, investigations, and program evaluations, OIG reduces the incidence of fraud, waste, abuse, and mismanagement, and promotes economy, efficiency, and effectiveness throughout DHHS. OIG is responsible for maintaining public confidence in the Medicare program and does so in the following manner:

- Agents investigate complaints that appear to be serious fraud or abuse and refer some cases to the Medicare carriers and/or intermediaries for initial work-up and review.

- OIG minimizes opportunities for fraud and abuse by recommending claims processing safeguards to HCFA and by investigating and helping to prosecute persons who violate regulations.

- OIG publicizes such prosecutions to deter similar actions by other individuals.

- OIG prepares cases that cannot be prosecuted as criminal complaints for civil prosecution under the Civil Monetary Penalties Act.

- OIG acts as a conduit for complaints from the public (via the OIG Hotline), Social Security offices, and other government entities.

The Office of Investigations (OI)

The OIG supervises investigations through its Office of Investigations (OI). This is staffed by professional criminal investigators. It has responsibility for all criminal investigations, including but not limited to Medicare fraud.

The OI presents cases in which a pattern of fraud has been documented to the Department of Justice for appropriate action. The OI is also responsible for developing and negotiating civil monetary penalty cases and for developing and implementing administrative sanctions against physicians and other providers for fraudulent or abusive activities.

The OI maintains field offices, called Office of Investigations Field Offices (OIFO), throughout the United States so they can be in closer contact to the carriers in their jurisdiction.

Office of Audit Services

A department of OIG, the Office of Audit Services conducts comprehensive audits to promote economy and efficiency and to prevent and detect fraud, abuse, and waste in operations and programs.

Office of Evaluation and Inspection

The role of this office is to identify program vulnerability to fraud, abuse, and waste. This is done by conducting inspections, evaluating the results, and making recommendations to improve the program's efficiency, effectiveness, and integrity.

Peer Review Organizations (PRO)

The Tax Equity and Fiscal Responsibility Act of 1982 (TEFRA '82) gave PROs authority to scrutinize the utilization and quality of services provided by hospitals, other health care institutions, and physicians. PROs insure that services are:

- Provided economically and only when and to the extent that they are medically necessary.

- Of a quality that meets professionally recognized standards of health care.

- Supported by the appropriate evidence of medical necessity and quality, in the form and fashion that the reviewing PRO may reasonably require (including copies of the necessary documentation) to assure that the provider is meeting these obligations.

Physicians and other providers who are suspected of violating these conditions are reviewed by a PRO. PROs make recommendations regarding providers' actions and forward the report to the OIG. The OIG then decides if sanctions or fines should be levied.

Contractors

Contractors—the carriers and intermediaries that contract with HCFA to provide administrative services—are given primary responsibility for identifying and developing cases of suspected fraud or abuse. These are then referred to the appropriate OIFO.

Contractors maintain a Program Safeguard Unit. This has responsibility for controlling and developing potential fraud and abuse cases within the Medicare program. The Program Safeguard staff includes professionals and trained assistants with extensive backgrounds in medicine, law enforcement, and claims examination.

This unit works closely with a number of different departments, public groups, and government agencies. Some of these include HCFA, OIG, the General Accounting Office (GAO), Assistant U.S. Attorneys, the Federal Bureau of Investigations (FBI), the Department of Justice, state medical boards, and various senior service organizations, such as American Association of Retired Persons.

The primary purpose of the Program Safeguard Unit is to identify cases of suspected fraud and abuse, and to refer them to the OIFO to be considered for criminal prosecution, civil prosecution, and/or administrative action. Other responsibilities include: training of internal and external departments and/or entities; safeguarding claims history; internal monitoring; and establishing communications about possible fraudulent or abusive activities.

One of the departments the Program Safeguard Unit works closely with is the Medical Review (MR) Unit. The

MR Unit's responsibility is to look for questionable billing patterns and practices, i.e., program abuse. HCFA believes that the Part B program is most vulnerable to overutilization of services.

The MR Unit helps detect and develop abuse cases primarily through analysis of claims data. Each provider's pattern of services is developed and analyzed and then compared against a norm. An "educational contact" is made to those who deviate from the norm. This contact describes the problem behavior detected and asks the provider to please correct it. Failure on the part of the provider to fix the problem can lead to a fraud investigation.

In addition, the Program Safeguard Unit has responsibility for initiating and conducting beneficiary and provider outreach programs. These programs include educating the public about potential areas of fraud and abuse and what to do if fraud or abuse is found. In addition to meeting with state and local consumer advocacy groups, provider and supplier associations, and beneficiary groups, the Program Safeguard Unit also publishes and sends to providers information in bulletins and educational pamphlets.

SOURCES OF LEADS

Medicare has many ways of generating fraud and abuse leads. Some of the sources for fraud leads are listed in Section 14004.1 of the *Medicare Carrier's Manual* and include:

• Reports from the General Accounting Office, Congressional committees, OIG Office of Audit Services, OIG Office of Investigations, or other oversight organizations at the federal, state, or local level.

- Suggestions from HCFA components, state agencies, contractors, and PROs, concerning areas where they have experienced problems or identified program matters that do not seem to be properly addressed in current policy.

- Statistical leads indicating aberrant costs, upcoding, or charging practices produced by state and contractor postpayment systems or other sources.

- Newspaper and magazine articles, as well as local and national television and radio programs highlighting areas of possible mismanagement or abuse.

- Carrier quality assurance (QA) staff.

- Complaints or questions from providers, beneficiaries, recipients, or private citizens.

- OIFO and HCFA fraud alerts.

- Investigative leads from ongoing fraud and abuse case review activity.

- Ideas stemming from ongoing or completed inspections.

In addition to the above, carriers use other resources to produce abuse leads. Some of these include:

- Referrals from other agencies, such as the Social Security Administration, the OIG, and HCFA Regional Offices.

- Complaints from beneficiaries and providers' employees. The Medicare program offers "rewards" to individuals who turn in a provider whom they believe is committing fraud or abuse.

- The carrier's staff, including the departments of program integrity; beneficiary services or medical correspondence; hearings; quality assurance; claims processing; provider/ professional relations; and private business.

- State Medicaid medical review results.

- Other carriers that may also serve physicians operating in the same territory.

- Questionable advertising by a provider, physician, or other supplier in local media.

- Newspaper accounts of a provider's, physician's, or supplier's prosecution.

- Mail returned as undeliverable.

- Postpayment review, a process used by carriers to detect payment errors made in the initial claims processing cycle and to detect inappropriate billing and practice patterns of physicians.

The OIG compiles statistical data on the sources for successful fraud prosecutions. Carriers as a source are followed closely by private citizens, which includes beneficiaries.

Medicare, through the OIG, sends informational pamphlets to beneficiaries to inform them of inappropriate arrangements, such as routine waiver of copayments and joint ventures. Statements about fraud and abuse are printed on EOMBs to encourage beneficiaries to report any suspected wrongdoing.

Beneficiaries are often considered the most reliable source of information for the development of fraud and abuse cases. However, as you learned earlier in this chapter, complaints can be generated due to misunderstandings of the billing process or of medical terminology. Former employees of offenders also make a strong contribution to the detection of cases. Complaints by former employees are usually taken very seriously as they are considered very reliable.

IF YOU SUSPECT A PROBLEM

You may be positive there is a problem if:

- Services were provided on dates when you were not in the city where the services were provided.

- Services were provided in a town where you have never been.

- Services billed were for services you are certain you did not have, such as a surgery or an office visit.

- Services billed were in excess of the number you received, such as four office visits in one week, when you only went to the office once.

- Services billed were for services other than the type you actually received, such as an emergency department visit when you saw the physician in his office.

- Hospital charges were from a hospital in a town other than yours.

- Hospital charges were for dates when you were not in the city where the services were provided.

- Charges were from a laboratory when you have not had any lab work performed.

- Charges were for medical equipment when your physician has not ordered any for you or you have not attempted to purchase or rent any.

- Instances where a supplier advertises or otherwise offers free medical equipment that your doctor did not prescribe.

- Charges were for outpatient services when you were an inpatient in the hospital.

- Charges were for home medical equipment when you were an inpatient in a hospital or skilled nursing facility (SNF).

- Charges were for ambulance services that you did not receive.

- Instances where a physician tells you that he can obtain Medicare payment for services that are considered noncovered.

- Instances where a clinic or doctor's office advertises free screening services and asks for your HICN or Medicare card. (If the services are free, why do they need your Medicare number?)

- Instances where a physician or other provider advertises or otherwise notifies all Medicare patients that they do not have to pay the coinsurance or deductible or that the practice will accept "insurance only."

If you are not completely positive, it is important to first identify whether there is a legitimate problem. Before contacting your carrier with a complaint, attempt to get an explanation from your physician's office. They may be able to explain a complicated billing matter or clarify why a service was billed in the way it was billed.

If their reply is satisfactory and makes sense to you, you may assume that you misunderstood. If they seem to hedge and do not provide a satisfactory response (or you cannot contact them because the number has been disconnected), you could assume that there is a problem and you may want to report it to the local carrier.

Also, keep a good record of services you receive, including the dates, place of service (e.g., office, hospital, emergency department), town, and type of service provided. Include also when your physician orders services for you, such as lab work or X-rays. This record may help you recall services you may have forgotten about—or help you identify services you did not receive.

Notify the Program Safeguards Department

If you suspect fraud or abuse, contact the fraud and abuse department of your local carrier. Many carriers and intermediaries have changed the name of their fraud and abuse departments to the Program Safeguards Department, partly because the departments are now working more proactively to prevent fraud and abuse and thus "safeguard" the Medicare program.

You can contact this department by calling or writing. The address and phone number are provided on the EOMB and in Appendix A of this book.

You do not have to give your name when you file a complaint. However, if you want to be notified of the outcome of the department's investigation, you will need to give your name, address, and Medicare number. When you call or write, be sure to include the following information:

1. Clear statement that you are filing a fraud or abuse complaint.

2. Provider's name and PIN. The PIN, or provider identification number, is provided on the EOMB by the provider's name and may also be listed as the PIN or Medicare number on the itemized bill (superbill) you received from the doctor.

3. The item or service in question.

4. The date on which the service is shown to have been furnished.

5. The amount approved and paid by Medicare.

6. The date of the EOMB.

7. The name and HICN of the person whom the EOMB indicates received the item or service.

8. The reason(s) you are questioning the Medicare payment for the item or service (e.g., "I was not in this town on the date of the service").

Once your complaint is received, the carrier is required to acknowledge it within 30 days. The Program Safeguards Department will give you a date by which they expect to complete their investigation of your complaint. If this is not possible, the department will give you a progress report every 60 days until the case is completed.

When the investigation is completed, a decision will be made by the investigator. In many cases, it is found that the provider correctly filed the claim and the services were legitimate, although they did not seem so to you. In this case, the investigator can explain the charges to you. In other cases, an honest billing mistake may have been made and the provider will correct it, including making any required refunds to you or to Medicare.

In cases where your complaint was accurate and the provider appears to have filed a fraudulent claim, the Medicare carrier will refer the case to the OIFO or OIG for civil, criminal, and/or administrative action. If you are told that the matter was referred to the OIG, that means that Medicare believes that fraud exists and that further criminal investigation is warranted.

Be aware that these types of investigations can be lengthy, taking many months or even years to complete.

Also, the carrier may not be able to provide you with detailed information if sensitive matters, including patient confidentiality, are involved. Know, however, that your complaint was appreciated and that you helped stop illegal—and expensive—activities.

INVESTIGATION AND DEVELOPMENT OF CASES

Fraud Cases

The OIG (through the OIFO) has authority to perform full-scale investigations and to levy sanctions and fines in fraud cases. However, carriers are responsible for completing the major portion of the initial investigation and development before referring cases to the OIFO. This section outlines the carrier's responsibility in developing fraud cases.

After receiving a complaint, the carrier begins to investigate the provider's background (e.g., past complaints, past warning letters for similar violations). Then research is done on the types of services involved, the provider's claims activity, prior identification on the Provider Audit List, and any other data that would indicate that the provider is intentionally defrauding the program.

Carriers are instructed to look carefully at the information to ascertain whether the provider has made a billing error or if he is truly attempting to commit a fraudulent act. If the carrier determines that no fraud has occurred, it will contact the provider to discuss the complaint with him. If necessary, the carrier educates the provider to help prevent any future occurrences.

While no penalties or other sanctions are levied, a summary of the case is still sent to the OIFO. If another complaint is received about the same physician, the carrier and the OIFO will use this information to make a determination regarding the current complaint.

Abuse Cases

The initial responsibility for investigating and correcting abuse rests with the carrier. The difference between a fraud investigation and an abuse investigation is essentially that an abuse situation involves a review of the medical necessity of the services billed, where a fraud investigation attempts to determine if the billed services were actually rendered.

In an abuse investigation, the carrier uses the same type of information that is used in fraud investigations: past billing history, prior identification for similar situations, etc. However, the focus is on utilization and the medical necessity of the services. Because of this, the carrier can request that a PRO, in addition to its own medical review staff, review the claims in question.

In situations where the carrier's actions are not effective in correcting the problem, the carrier will refer the case to the HCFA Regional Office, because in some cases, failure by the provider to correct a problem changes the classification from abuse to fraud. This applies in three situations: violation of the assignment agreement, violation of the participation agreement, and violation of the limiting charge.

If a physician breaches the assignment agreement, the carrier will contact him, in person, by phone, and/or by mail. The physician must assure the carrier that any amounts collected in error will be refunded and that there will be no further violations. The state or local medical society may be enlisted to help the carrier obtain the necessary assurances from the physician.

After this contact, the physician will receive a follow-up letter detailing the assignment obligations. If the physician "cleans up his act" and makes no further violations, the case is closed. If, however, the physician fails to correct the problem, the case will be referred to the HCFA Regional Office for further action.

The Regional Office can revoke the physician's assignment privilege and levy fines. If the physician violates the assignment agreement after receiving a warning, he is *willfully and intentionally* violating the regulations. Consequently, the case is referred to the OIFO, which then considers whether to recommend criminal prosecution or civil penalties and/or revoke the physician's assignment privilege.

The same basic rules apply to violations of the participation agreement and of limiting charges. If the violation was an error, the physician has the opportunity to correct it. If, after a warning from the carrier, the physician makes the same violations, the case will be referred to the OIFO and investigated for fraud.

SANCTIONS AND PENALTIES

Medicare has authority under the law to "punish" providers who violate the regulations. These "punishments" take the form of administrative sanctions: revocation of assignment privileges and withholding of benefit payments; fines; civil penalties, such as exclusion from the Medicare program; and criminal charges. The sanction is different depending upon the type and frequency of the violation.

Sanctions

Carriers (as well as other agencies of HCFA) have the authority to impose administrative sanctions. Administrative sanctions are designed to encourage the provider to correct his behavior. They are used only to correct abuse; fraud can carry civil and criminal penalties. A brief explanation of the procedure for each type of sanction is provided below.

Educational Contact and/or Warning: Before doing anything else, the carrier contacts the physician, explaining that a violation has occurred, why the action is considered a violation, that it must be corrected, and how to correct the problem. This initial contact also includes a warning that if the physician persists in committing this violation, more serious penalties could result.

Withholding of Payments/Recovery of Overpayments: When the carrier determines that an overpayment has occurred, a decision is made whether to withhold future Medicare payments. In cases of abuse, the physician is usually notified prior to the suspension of payment and provided an opportunity to submit additional evidence to refute the determination. In cases of possible fraud, payment is suspended prior to notifying the physician.

Revocation of Assignment Privileges: A provider's assignment privileges are revoked in more serious situations, such as repeated violations of the assignment agreement. Revocation is used to deny payment while criminal prosecution is being considered or is in process. It may also be appropriate when prosecution is not feasible.

Referral of Situations to State Licensing Boards or Medical/Professional Societies: In instances of apparent unethical or improper practices or unprofessional conduct, the carrier can refer the case to state licensing authorities, medical boards, a PRO, or professional societies for review and possible disciplinary action.

Exclusion

Physicians and other individuals who have been convicted of fraudulent activities against Medicare or other state health care programs may be excluded from participation in the Medicare program. This authority was granted to the Secretary of DHHS by the Medicare and Medicaid Patient and Program Protection Act of 1987. The Secretary transfers this authority to the OIG.

Exclusion from participation does not mean that the provider can submit bills as a nonparticipating provider. An excluded provider cannot render care to any patient who receives Medicare benefits. He cannot bill the program at all. A provider who is excluded from Medicare is also automatically excluded from participation in state programs, such as Medicaid, Maternal and Child Health Services, and Social Service Block Grants.

A provider can be excluded from the program if he has: (1) submitted bills or requests for payment that contain charges for items or services furnished substantially in excess of his usual charges; (2) furnished items or services to patients that are substantially in excess of the needs of such patients; or (3) furnished items or services to patients that are of a quality that does not meet professionally recognized standards of health care.

In addition to excluding providers from participation in the program, the OIG has also been empowered to exclude from coverage items and services rendered by providers who have engaged in certain forms of program abuse. Examples of abuse cases that can be considered for program exclusion include, but are not limited to:

- Providers who have been the subject of an adverse peer review finding.

- Providers whose bills must be reviewed continually because of repeated instances of overutilization.

- Providers who furnish or cause to be furnished items or services that are substantially in excess of the patient's needs or are of a quality that does not meet professionally recognized standards of health care.

- Providers who are the subject of prepayment review for an extended period of time (longer than six months) and who have not corrected their pattern of practice after receiving educational/warning letters.

Generally, to be excluded for abuse, a provider must demonstrate a pattern of consistent refusal or failure to remedy the situation in spite of efforts on the part of the carrier to help the provider correct the problem.

A provider who is being considered for exclusion has appeal rights available. If the provider is finally excluded, the OIG notifies HCFA, the carrier, the state Medicaid program, the PRO, the Railroad Retirement Board, the appropriate licensing agency, the public (through a newspaper notice), and all known employees of the sanctioned provider. If a beneficiary presents a claim for benefits after the date of the exclusion, the beneficiary will be notified at that time that the provider has been excluded from the program and *payment will not be made to the beneficiary.*

Criminal Charges

The Medicare program, through the OIG, has the authority to make criminal charges against providers who violate the regulations. Many cases of fraud are prosecuted as felonies. Some cases of abuse, especially those types where the provider has refused to comply with requests to rectify a problem, can also carry criminal charges. Examples of situations for which a provider may be criminally charged are shown in Figure 8-1.

Fines

The OIG has authority to levy fines against providers for fraud and abuse. Typically, the fines include refund of any overpayments made, plus interest, plus a charge for committing the fraud or abuse.

Figure 8-1: Actions Carrying Criminal Charges and the Penalties

Offense	Maximum Allowable Penalty
Soliciting or receiving a bribe, kickback, or rebate. This includes routine waiver of coinsurance and deductibles. (Felony)	$25,000 fine 5 years imprisonment Exclusion (min. 5 years)
Unlicensed or fraudulently licensed physician presenting a claim for physician's service. Includes claims for a physician's services that were actually rendered by auxillary personnel not under the direct personal supervision of the physician. (Felony)	$25,000 fine 5 years imprisonment Exclusion (min. 5 years)
Racketeering. Any activity or threat involving: murder, kidnaping, gambling, arson, robbery, extortion or dangerous drugs; also bankruptcy fraud or securities fraud. (Felony)	$25,000 fine 20 years imprisonment Exclusion (min. 5 years)
Presenting fictitious or fraudulent claims, including billing for services not rendered, misrepresentation of services rendered, application for duplicate reimbursement. (Felony or Misdemeanor)	$10,000 fine 5 years imprisonment Exclusion (min. 5 years)
Possession of false papers with intent to defraud. (Felony)	$10,000 fine 5 years imprisonment Exclusion (min. 5 years)

Figure 8-1 *(continued)*: Criminal Charges and the Penalties

Offense	Maximum Allowable Penalty
Making false statements or concealing facts during an investigation. (Felony)	$10,000 fine 5 years imprisonment Exclusion (min. 5 years)
Obstruction of audit or investigation process by concealing, destroying, altering, etc., requested records. (Felony)	$5,000 fine 5 years imprisonment Exclusion (min. 5 years)
Mail fraud. (Felony)	$1,000 fine 5 years imprisonment Exclusion (min. 5 years)
Making a false statement to qualify as a provider. (Misdemeanor)	$2,000 fine 6 months imprisonment Exclusion (min. 5 years)
Making false representations to anyone concerning the program. (Misdemeanor)	$1,000 fine 1 year imprisonment Exclusion (min. 5 years)
Deceiving, misleading, or threatening a claimant by word, letter, or advertisement. (Misdemeanor)	$500 fine 1 year imprisonment Exclusion (min.5 years)
Forging or altering public or legal documents; publishing or presenting such altered documents as true (Felony)	$1,000 fine 10 years imprisonment Exclusion (min. 5 years)
Repeated violation of assignment agreement. (Misdemeanor)	$2,000 fine 6 months imprisonment Exclusion (min. 5 years)

The Medicare and Medicaid Patient and Program Protection Act of 1987—sometimes called the Civil Monetary Penalty Law (CMPL)—gave authority to the Secretary of DHHS to impose civil monetary penalties for violations of program regulations. The amount of the penalty is *in addition* to any overpayments and interest amounts the provider may be required to repay. Depending upon the violation, different penalties apply. Violations are described below.

Preparing, Presenting or Causing to Be Presented, or Submitting False or Fictitious Claims

Note that this category includes "causing to be presented." This clause could include the provider who "looks the other way" or encourages the behavior by saying nothing without actually getting involved. Just because the provider isn't actually completing the form does not mean he will not be considered party to the violation. Some examples of the types of activities that could fall under this category are:

- Billing for no-shows.

- Upcoding.

- Billing for services that were not furnished at all, such as charges for hospital visits when the physician was on vacation.

- Billing for nonphysician services for services of practitioners who are not under the direct personal supervision of the physician or while the physician is out of town.

- Altering medical records, either by adding or deleting information.

- Unbundling.

- Claims that include or are supported by false or fraudulent records.

- Billing for supplies that do not represent a cost to the physician.

- Billing Medicare for primary benefits when Medicare is the secondary payer.

- Including diagnoses on claims just to obtain reimbursement, for example, listing bladder tumors just to obtain reimbursement for a cystoscopy.

Presenting Claims in Violation of the Assignment Agreement or the Participation Agreement

Some examples of the types of activities that could fall under this category are:

- Billing or charging patients for completing or filing claim forms.

- Failure to accept assignment for clinical diagnostic laboratory tests.

- Failure to accept assignment for a Medicaid-eligible Medicare beneficiary.

- Failure to accept assignment for services of certain auxiliary personnel (e.g., nurse-practitioners and physician assistants).

- Collecting more than Medicare's allowable (except in some secondary payer situations).

- Billing patients for services denied as not reasonable and necessary (unless the patient was notified in writing in advance of the possibility of denial and the patient signed a written agreement to pay).

- Failure by a participating provider to accept assignment.

- An attempt by a participating provider to collect more than the copayment and deductible from the patient.

- Billing more than the limiting charge on unassigned claims.

- Failure by a nonparticipating provider to provide advance notice to the patient for unassigned claims for elective surgery costing more than $500.

- Failure to make a refund to the patient within 30 days for unassigned claims for services denied as not reasonable and necessary.

- An attempt to mark-up purchased diagnostic tests.

Omission of Information

Some examples of the types of activities that could fall under this category are:

- Failure to include ICD-9-CM diagnosis codes.

- Failure to include referring physician information.

- Failure to include outside supplier information for purchased diagnostic tests.

- Repeated failure to include pertinent claims information, such as assignment acknowledgment, the physician's signature, primary payer information, etc.

- Failure to include appropriate HCPCS codes (including CPT and national codes).

- Failure by the physician to report ownership arrangements he may have with other entities.

- Failure to include payments made by the patient.

- Failure to report liability or settlement payments.

As you can see, the law has gone to great lengths to protect the Medicare program, and its beneficiaries, from the costs of fraud and abuse. While many providers are honest and caring, a few take advantage of the system. It is important to be aware of this, and to be educated and knowledgeable about activities that constitute fraud and abuse, so that you can help in the detection of these activities.

CHAPTER 9

MEDICARE AS SECONDARY PAYER

Medicare as secondary payer (MSP) refers to situations where Medicare pays benefits only after another insurer—the primary payer—makes a determination on the claim. This provision is similar to *coordination of benefits* used for commercial health insurance. MSP is often very confusing to beneficiaries, who believe that Medicare pays for their medical care "no matter what." This is not true: many laws have been passed identifying different types of insurance that must pay benefits primary to Medicare.

As you have learned in previous chapters, the health care provider is responsible for submitting claims for services provided to you. Since you are the only person who knows what kind of health insurance coverage you have, it is very important that you notify your physician or the hospital if:

- You work and have group health insurance from your employer.

- Your spouse works and you are covered on your spouse's group health insurance.

- Your treatment is needed due to an injury or illness caused by your job.

- Your treatment is needed due to a car accident.

- Your treatment is needed due to an injury that occurred on property that belongs to another person or company.

- You have end stage renal disease (ESRD) and are/were employed and have group health insurance from your employer or your spouse's employer.

- You are disabled and have group health insurance from your employer or your spouse's employer.

- Your treatment is needed due to an illness caused by your work in a coal mine.

- You are a veteran.

In the cases listed above, Medicare is responsible for paying only secondary benefits. Under MSP law, there are six categories for which Medicare pays secondary benefits; they are:

- Working aged and spouses

- Workers' Compensation

- Disabled

- ESRD

- Automobile medical and no-fault

- Liability

This chapter describes each category by providing a general overview, including pertinent definitions, describing to whom the provision applies, and outlining when conditional primary payments might be made.

IDENTIFYING MSP SITUATIONS

In all cases, Medicare makes every effort to "mark" those beneficiaries for whom another insurer may be primary. One important method Medicare uses to help the carriers and intermediaries identify potential MSP situations is the MSP Data Match Program, which is an information network among different government agencies. Some of the agencies involved in the MSP Data Match Program are:

- State Workers' Compensation agencies.

- Other third-party payers.

- Internal Revenue Service (IRS).

As part of its pairing with the IRS, the Health Care Financing Administration (HCFA) sends questionnaires to a sample of employers. In this way they obtain information about employees and their spouses who are eligible for Medicare and who participate in employer group health plans. Employers who fail to respond promptly and accurately to these questionnaires can face civil monetary penalties.

Also, when you sign up for Social Security benefits or Medicare benefits, you are asked whether you are working and whether you have insurance through your employer or your spouse's employer. Persons who do not tell the truth regarding their coverage can face fraud charges.

Another way contractors identify beneficiaries with other coverage is by "screening" claims when they are submitted. Medicare "catches" these claims as part of its normal processing procedures by checking whether:

- The work-related questions on the claim form (Items 8 and/or 10a of the HCFA-1500) are answered "yes."

- The health insurance claim form (Item 10b of the HCFA-1500) shows that the services were related to an automobile or other accident.

- Items 9 or 11 of the HCFA-1500 form indicates that the individual is employed and covered under a group health plan or is the spouse of an employee and is covered under the spouse's group health plan or that these items indicate another insurer.

- The beneficiary previously received benefits from another insurer for the same condition or a claim for such benefits is pending.

- The claim shows as complementary insurer an insurance organization that does not issue health insurance.

- The diagnosis is one that is commonly associated with employment, e.g., pneumoconiosis; radiation sickness; anthrax; undulant fever; dermatitis due to contact with industrial compounds; lead, arsenic, or mercury poisoning.

- There is indication that the injury or illness occurred on the job.

- The patient has been identified as a Federal Black Lung or Workers' Compensation beneficiary.

- Information from a physician, beneficiary, a carrier's Medicare or private insurance staff, another Medicare contractor, or any other source indicates that Medicare has been billed for services when there is a possibility of payment by another insurer.

- The carrier (or the HCFA Regional Office) is asked to endorse a check from a no-fault insurer payable to Medicare and the beneficiary.

- The carrier receives or is informed of a request from an insurance company or from an attorney for copies of bills or medical records.

- The carrier receives an ambulance claim indicating that trauma-related services were involved and the claim does not provide a specific point of origin (i.e., a residential street address).

If the carrier determines that other coverage might exist, a letter is sent to the claimant instructing him to submit the claim to the primary insurer and, after that insurer makes its determination, to resubmit the claim to Medicare for secondary benefits.

A claim for services that includes the primary payer's determination is processed for secondary benefits. The primary payer's decision to pay or deny a claim is not binding on the Medicare carrier. Medicare is not required to follow the guidelines of the primary payer in relation to medical necessity, coverage of services, etc. However, if the primary payer pays only for certain services either because the plan does not cover those services or because benefits available under the plan have been exhausted, Medicare may pay primary benefits for those services, provided they are otherwise covered by Medicare.

DEVELOPMENT

If a claim is received and the contractor cannot identify the primary payer's determination, the contractor "develops" the claim. This means the contractor will contact the involved parties to obtain answers to questionable items.

If the Medicare claim is not accompanied by the primary payer's Explanation of Benefits (EOB), the claim will be returned to the claimant with instructions that the EOB must be submitted before the secondary claim can be processed. If the primary payer's EOB does not include needed information, or contains information that is inconsistent with the Medicare claim (for example, the physician's name, date of service, charges, etc., are different on the primary claim), the carrier will ask the primary payer for the information. If the information cannot be obtained from the primary payer, the Medicare carrier will contact the beneficiary and/or the physician for assistance in developing the claim.

If the primary payer's allowable charge information is not included, the Medicare carrier will process the claim based on the assumption that the physician's actual charge on the claim is the primary payer's allowable. Benefits will be paid accordingly.

If a contractor contacts you for information related to a claim, provide all the requested information and return it as quickly as possible. Failure to provide accurate information could be considered fraud.

CALCULATING SECONDARY BENEFITS

When Secondary Benefits Are Payable

Medicare may pay secondary benefits when a provider, physician, supplier, or beneficiary bills a third party payer for primary benefits and that payer does not pay the entire charge for the items or services, and the provider, physician, or supplier does not accept, and is not obligated to accept, the payment as full payment.

What does this mean? Medicare may make a payment beyond what the primary payer paid if the provider or physician is not obligated to accept that payer's payment as payment in full. For example, most state Workers' Compensation laws stipulate that payment made by Workers' Compensation for medical services constitutes full discharge of the patient's liability for payment of the services. This means that the hospital or physician is obligated to accept the Workers' Compensation payment as payment in full, and so no secondary Medicare benefits would be payable.

Conversely, payment made by an employer's group health insurer typically does not constitute full payment (unless the provider accepted assignment). If this amount is less than Medicare's allowable for the service, Medicare may pay secondary benefits.

Application of Deductible Amounts

Expenses for Medicare-covered services that are paid for by a third party payer are credited toward the Medicare Part A and Part B deductibles.

Utilization

Because Medicare is making a payment toward covered services, even though it is not the primary payer of these services, it keeps track of the number of days of inpatient hospital care used by a beneficiary. This is called utilization of inpatient days. This calculation is used to help determine the beneficiary's liability for charges. The rules for calculating utilization are as follows:

- If the days resulting from the utilization calculation are fewer than the full days available for the stay, no coinsurance days are billed.

- If the days resulting from the utilization calculation are greater than the full days available for the stay, coinsurance days are billed for the excess days.

For example, a beneficiary has 17 full days available at admission. The hospital stay was 20 days. After performing the calculation to determine the chargeable utilization, it is determined that the beneficiary can be charged with 10 days. Since the beneficiary did not exceed the remaining days left in the benefit period before coinsurance could be charged, the beneficiary will not be liable for payment of coinsurance.

As another example, a beneficiary has used 60 days of a benefit period and was admitted to the hospital during the same benefit period. This means he has 30 "coinsurance days" available before being required to use lifetime reserve days. The hospital stay was 20 days. After performing the calculation to determine the chargeable utilization, it is determined that the beneficiary can be charged with 10 days. Therefore, only 10 coinsurance days are billed to the beneficiary.

Inpatient psychiatric hospital and skilled nursing facility care that is paid for by a third party payer is not counted against the number of inpatient care days available to the beneficiary under Medicare Part A.

Calculating Secondary Benefits

Part A

For Part A covered services, the Medicare secondary payment is the lowest of:

1. The gross amount payable by Medicare minus the applicable deductible and coinsurance amounts.

2. The gross amount payable by Medicare minus the amount paid by the primary insurer.

3. The provider's charges (or the amount the provider is obligated to accept as payment in full, if that is less than the charges) minus the amount payable by the primary insurer.

4. The provider's charges (or the amount the provider is obligated to accept as payment in full, if that is less than the charges) minus the applicable Medicare deductible and coinsurance amounts.

The gross amount payable by Medicare is the gross amount payable by Medicare without considering the effect of the Medicare deductible and coinsurance amounts or the payment by the primary payer.

To better understand how Medicare calculates secondary payment for Part A services, consider four examples.

Example One:

Local Hospital furnished 7 days of inpatient hospital care in 1996 to a Medicare beneficiary. The provider's charges for Medicare-covered services totaled $2,800. The primary insurer paid $2,360. No part of the Medicare inpatient deductible of $736 had been met. If the gross amount payable by Medicare would have been $2,700, then as secondary payer, Medicare pays the lowest of:

1. The gross amount payable by Medicare minus the hospital inpatient deductible: $2,700 — $736 = $1,964.

2. The gross amount payable by Medicare minus the amount paid by the primary insurer: $2,700 — $2,360 = $340.

3. The provider's charges minus the amount paid by the primary insurer: $2,800 — $2,360 = $440.

4. The provider's charges minus the inpatient hospital deductible: $2,800 — $736 = $2,064.

Medicare's secondary payment is $340. The combined payments made by the primary insurer and Medicare total $2,700. The $736 deductible was satisfied by the primary insurer's payment of $2,360, so the beneficiary has no out-of-pocket expense.

Example Two:

A hospital furnished 1 day of inpatient hospital care in 1996 to a Medicare beneficiary. The provider's charges for Medicare-covered services totaled $750. The primary insurer paid $450. No part of the hospital inpatient deductible had been met previously. The primary insurer's payment is credited toward the Medicare hospital inpatient deductible. If the gross amount payable by Medicare in this case would have been $850, then as secondary payer, Medicare pays the lowest of:

1. The gross amount payable by Medicare minus the deductible: $850 — $736 = $114.

2. The gross amount payable by Medicare minus the amount paid by the primary insurer: $850 — $450 = $400.

3. The provider's charges minus the amount paid by the primary insurer: $750 — $450 = $300.

4. The provider's charges minus the Medicare deductible: $750 — $736 = $14.

Medicare will pay $14. The combined payment made by the primary insurer and Medicare totaled $464. The beneficiary's liability is $286 (the $736 deductible minus the $450 primary insurer payment). This is the amount the hospital can charge the beneficiary.

Example Three:

A hospital furnished five days of inpatient care in 1996 to a Medicare beneficiary. No part of the hospital inpatient deductible of $736 had been met. The hospital's charges for Medicare-covered services were $4,000 and the Medicare gross amount payable would have been $3,500. The provider agreed to accept $3,000 as payment in full. The primary payer paid $2,900 to satisfy its $100 deductible requirement. Medicare considers the amount the provider is obligated to accept ($3,000) as the hospital's charges in this situation. As secondary payer, Medicare pays the lowest of:

1. The gross amount payable by Medicare minus the deductible: $3,500 — $736 = $2,764.

2. The gross amount payable by Medicare minus the amount paid by the primary insurer: $3,500 — $2,900 = $600.

3. The provider's charges minus the amount paid by the primary insurer: $3,000 — $2,900 = $100.

4. The provider's charges minus the Medicare deductible: $3,000 — $736 = $2,264.

Medicare will pay $100. The combined payment made by the primary insurer and Medicare totaled $3,000. The beneficiary has no liability since the primary insurer's payment satisfied the $736 inpatient deductible.

Example Four:

A hospital furnished 20 days of inpatient hospital care to a Medicare beneficiary, all of which were lifetime reserve days. The hospital's charges were $4,000. The inpatient hospital deductible had been met previously. The primary insurer paid $2,400 for Medicare covered services. The gross amount payable by Medicare would have been $3,700. As secondary payer, Medicare pays the lowest of:

1. The gross amount payable by Medicare minus the coinsurance amount ($184 x 20 days):
   $3,700 — $3,680 = $20.

2. The gross amount payable by Medicare minus the amount paid by the primary insurer:
   $3,700 — $2,400 = $1,300.

3. The provider's charges minus the amount paid by the primary insurer: $4,000 — $2,400 = $1,600.

4. The provider's charges minus the Medicare coinsurance amount: $4,000 — $3,680 = $320.

Medicare will pay $20. Since the primary payer's payment ($2,400) is less than the coinsurance ($3,680), full utilization is charged and coinsurance is determined in the usual manner. The beneficiary's liability is $1,280 (the $3,680 coinsurance minus the primary insurer's payment of $2,400). This is the amount the hospital can charge the beneficiary.

Part B

The amount of secondary benefits payable for Part B services is the lowest of:

1. The actual charge by the physician or supplier (or the amount he is obligated to accept as payment in full, if that amount is less than the actual charge) minus the amount paid by the primary payer.

2. The amount Medicare would pay if it were the primary insurer.

3. The higher of the Medicare allowable or the third party payer's allowable minus the amount actually paid by the primary payer.

Medicare will pay the lowest of the amounts calculated in steps 1, 2, and 3.

Let's consider two examples. Mrs. Franklin received treatment from Dr. Jefferson for which he charged $1,000. The primary payer allowed $900 of the charge and paid 80 percent of its allowable, or $720. The Medicare allowable is $680. Mrs. Franklin has met her Part B deductible.

1. Calculate the actual charge by the physician or supplier (or the amount he is obligated to accept as payment in full, if that amount is less than the actual charge) minus the amount paid by the primary payer.

Actual charge:	$ 1,000
Amount paid:	— 720
Difference:	**= $ 280**

2. Calculate the amount Medicare would pay if it were the primary payer.

Medicare allowable:	$ 680
Less 20% coinsurance:	— 136
Amount Medicare would pay:	**= $ 544**

3. Determine the higher of the Medicare allowable or the primary payer's allowable minus the amount actually paid by the primary payer.

Primary payer's allowable:	$ 900
Medicare's allowable:	$ 680
Higher amount:	$ 900
Less amount paid by primary payer	— 720
Difference:	**= $ 180**

Medicare will pay the lowest of the amounts calculated in steps 1, 2, and 3.

Step 1 = $280
Step 2 = $544
Step 3 = $180

Medicare will pay an additional $180 to Dr. Jefferson.

As another example, Mrs. Roosevelt received treatment from Dr. Kennedy for which the doctor charged $150. Mrs. Roosevelt has not met her annual deductible of $100. The primary payer's allowable for the service is $110, of which the payer paid 80 percent, or $88. The Medicare allowable for this treatment is $120. Medicare's secondary payment is calculated as follows:

1. Calculate the actual charge by the physician or supplier minus the amount paid by the primary payer.

Actual charge:	$ 150
Amount paid:	— 88
Difference:	**= $ 62**

2. Calculate the amount Medicare would pay if it were the primary payer.

Medicare allowable:	$ 120
Less unpaid deductible:	— 100
Remaining:	20
Less 20% coinsurance:	— 4
Amount Medicare would pay	**= $ 16**

3. Determine the higher of the Medicare allowable or the primary payer's allowable minus the amount actually paid by the primary payer.

Primary payer's allowable:	$ 110
Medicare's allowable:	$ 120
Higher amount:	$ 120
Less amount paid by primary payer:	— 88
Difference:	**= $ 32**

Medicare will pay the lowest of the amounts calculated in steps 1, 2, and 3.

   Step 1 = $ 62
   Step 2 = $ 16
   Step 3 = $ 32

Medicare will pay an additional $32 to Dr. Kennedy. Mrs. Roosevelt's Medicare deductible is credited with $100, which is the amount that would have been credited to the deductible based on the Medicare allowable of $120, if Medicare had been the primary payer. Mrs. Roosevelt owes Dr. Kennedy $100 for the amount of the deductible.

How Much Can the Physician Charge?

When another insurer pays benefits primary to Medicare, physicians are limited in the amount they are allowed to collect from the beneficiary. When the amount paid or payable by the primary insurer to the beneficiary exceeds the Medicare allowable (without regard to the coinsurance or deductible), the physician may retain the primary insurer's payment in full without violating the terms of assignment.

If the primary insurer's payment is less than the applicable Medicare deductible and coinsurance amounts, then the physician is limited to collecting the difference between the Medicare allowable (or the amount the physician is obligated to accept as payment in full, if less) and the sum of the primary insurer's payment and the Medicare secondary payment.

An example will help clarify this point. Dr. Jones charges $262 for a service. The primary payer allows $262 but pays only $112 because the beneficiary owes $150 deductible. The Medicare allowable is $200. The amount that Medicare pays as secondary payer is $80 since the Medicare secondary payment amount cannot exceed the amount Medicare would pay as primary payer.

$200 allowable — $100 Part B deductible = $100
$100 x 80 percent = $80 Medicare payment

The combined primary insurer payment and Medicare secondary payment is $192 ($112 + $80).

The physician may charge the beneficiary $8, which is the difference between the Medicare allowable ($200) and the sum of the primary insurer's payment and the Medicare secondary payment ($112 + $80 = $192). The $8 charge to the beneficiary represents the portion of the Part B deductible and coinsurance amounts in excess of the primary plan's payment.

The $100 Part B deductible is credited in full. The remaining $12 of the primary plan's payment is applied to the beneficiary's Part B coinsurance obligation of $20, leaving him responsible for the remaining coinsurance amount of $8.

Also, a physician may not collect more than the primary insurer's allowable when it is less than the Medicare allowable. In the second example above, Dr. Kennedy received $88 from the primary insurer and $32 from Medicare for a total of $110, which is the primary insurer's allowable amount. Even though Medicare's allowable is higher than the primary payer's allowable, he may not collect any more money from the patient; that is, he may not balance bill the patient. (The physician may, however, collect any unpaid portion of the patient's primary insurance or Medicare deductible.)

WORKING AGED AND SPOUSES

This category makes Medicare the secondary payer for individuals and their spouses who receive health insurance from an employer. For services rendered on or after January 1, 1983, Medicare is the secondary payer to an employer group health plan (EGHP) for Medicare-eligible persons who are working and who are over age 65 (working aged).

This category of MSP was extended to the spouses of working aged for services rendered on or after May 1, 1986.

Employers with 20 or more employees are required by the Age Discrimination in Employment Act to offer the same type of health insurance coverage to workers and their spouses who are over age 65 as they offer to workers and their spouses who are under age 65. The working aged employee may reject the employer's health plan, in which case Medicare is the primary payer. If the working aged employee rejects the employer's coverage, the employer *may not* offer secondary benefits. It is also against the law for an insurance plan to be written so it mandates that it will only pay secondary benefits if Medicare coverage is available. (For help in deciding whether to accept Medicare benefits or the EGHP benefits, see Chapter Five.)

Definitions

Employer: Individuals and organizations engaged in a trade or business and organizations exempt from income tax, such as religious, charitable, and educational institutions. Included are the governments of the United States, the individual states, the District of Columbia, the Virgin Islands, Guam, American Samoa, the Northern Mariana Islands, and Puerto Rico. (This provision applies only to employers with 20 or more full- or part-time employees. This requirement must be met at the time the individual receives the services for which Medicare benefits are claimed.)

Employed individual: Employees and self-employed persons such as directors of corporations and owners of businesses. If a self-employed individual enrolls in an EGHP that meets the definition of a plan (see below), the employer plan may be primary payer for that individual and the individual's spouse. Employed individuals also include members of the clergy and of religious orders who are reimbursed for their services by a church, religious order, or other employing entity.

Plan: Any arrangement by an employer, by more than one employer, or by an employee organization to provide health benefits or medical care to employees.

Employer Group Health Plan (EGHP): Any health plan that is provided by or contributed to by an employer of 20 or more employees that provides medical care directly or through insurance or reimbursement to current or former employees and/or their families. A plan that does not have any employees as enrollees, e.g., a plan for self-employed persons only, does not meet the definition of an EGHP. CHAMPUS does not meet the definition of an EGHP, however, the Federal Employees Health Benefits program does.

Note: Medicare is secondary to EGHP coverage only if the EGHP coverage is based on the covered person's current employment. Health insurance plans for retirees or the spouses of retirees do not meet this condition and are not primary to Medicare.

Secondary: Medicare is the secondary or residual payer to all EGHPs under which the Medicare beneficiary is covered by reason of current employment and will not pay for any expenses that are reimbursable by any such plan or plans.

To Whom the Provision Applies

Under the law, Medicare pays secondary benefits to an EGHP when the person meets the following conditions on the date the service was rendered:

- The patient is over age 65, is entitled to Medicare Part A and Part B, is employed, and as a result of that employment receives coverage under an EGHP.

- The patient is the spouse of an employed person, is over age 65, and is covered by the employed person's EGHP.

- The policy holder is actively working (not retired).

For instance, Mr. Adams works for the Widget Factory. He is entitled to Part A and Part B benefits and is also insured through his employer's group health insurance plan. In this case, the Widget Factory's plan is the primary insurer for Mr. Adams; Medicare pays only secondary benefits. Following this example, Mrs. Adams, a homemaker and Medicare beneficiary, also is insured on the Widget Factory's plan. In Mrs. Adams' case, Medicare would pay secondary benefits because she has other health insurance through her spouse's employer's plan.

Medicare is also secondary to an EGHP for self-employed individuals who are former employees if the employer provides coverage for other such individuals. The working aged and spouse provision does not apply:

- If the patient is entitled, or could be entitled upon application, to Medicare under the end-stage renal disease provision.

- To individuals enrolled in Part B only.

- To individuals enrolled in Part A on the basis of a monthly premium.

- To anyone who is under age 65.

- To individuals covered by a health plan other than an EGHP, e.g., one that is purchased by the individual privately and not as a member of a group.

- To employees of employers of fewer than 20 employees.

- To members of multi-employer plans whom the plan identified as employees of employers with fewer than 20 employees.

- To retired beneficiaries (other than spouses of employed individuals) who are covered by EGHPs as a result of past employment and who do not have EGHP coverage as the result of current employment.

The coordination period—the period when Medicare changes from secondary to primary payer—ceases on:

- The last day of the month in which the beneficiary or the beneficiary's spouse retires.

- The day the beneficiary or the beneficiary's spouse is terminated from the EGHP.

- The beneficiary's date of death.

Expenses paid by the EGHP count toward the Part B deductible and are credited up to the amount of Medicare's allowable for the service. For example, if the EGHP paid $75 for a service and Medicare's allowable for the service is $50, the beneficiary's deductible is credited $50—the amount of Medicare's allowable.

Conditional Primary Benefits

Conditional primary benefits refer to primary benefits paid by Medicare under an agreement that when the EGHP pays primary benefits, both the beneficiary and the EGHP are responsible for repaying the amount of the benefits to Medicare. Under the working aged and spouse provision, conditional primary benefits may be paid in only two situations:

1. The beneficiary has appealed or is protesting the EGHP denial of the claim for any reason other than the EGHP offers only secondary coverage of services covered by Medicare.

2. The EGHP denied the claim because the time limit for filing the claim with the EGHP has expired (whether appealed or not).

In the first situation, Medicare may make payment to the beneficiary. The carrier will then contact the employer plan to explain that the EGHP is obligated by law to pay primary benefits (even if the plan has collected premiums for secondary coverage only). The beneficiary will be notified by letter of the problem and advised to contact the insurer and the state insurance commission.

WORKERS' COMPENSATION

Workers' Compensation (WC) refers to state-administered programs that pay medical benefits to employees who are injured as a result of their employment or in the course of performing their duties on the job. Employers pay premiums to the WC agency based on the number and type of employees they employ. If an employee is injured in the course of performing his duties or as a result of his employment, WC is responsible for reimbursement for the necessary services.

Shortly after Medicare's inception, it became secondary payer to WC. Effective for services rendered on or after July 1, 1966, a Medicare-eligible individual who can reasonably expect to be reimbursed for services by WC can submit only claims for secondary benefits to Medicare.

The WC category also includes individuals who are entitled to federal Black Lung benefits. The Federal Black Lung Program is a government-sponsored program that allows coal miners and other individuals to receive benefits from the Department of Labor (DOL) for pneumocentesis caused by work in a coal mine. The Black Lung category became primary to Medicare for dates of service on or after July 1, 1973.

To Whom the Provision Applies

This category of MSP applies to any person who is entitled to Medicare and can claim WC or Black Lung benefits due to a job-related illness or injury. Note that WC or the DOL is responsible for payment of treatment related only to the job-related illness or injury or to the Black Lung disease; Medicare is responsible for primary payment for treatment for all other conditions. Medicare switches to primary payer on:

- The date the job-related illness or injury ceases or WC or Black Lung makes a settlement with the beneficiary.

- The beneficiary's date of death.

If the WC or Black Lung insurer is responsible for medical expenses related to the injury or illness for life, Medicare remains the secondary payer for the particular illness or injury. Medicare may pay primary benefits if the WC benefits are exhausted or if the beneficiary is in a category of noncovered employment.

Conditional Primary Payments

Medicare may make conditional payments pending a final decision on a WC claim. Conditional payments are made to avoid imposing hardship on a beneficiary while a decision is being made by the WC agency, since there is commonly a long delay between the occurrence of an injury and the WC decision. Conditional payments may be made in only two situations:

1. The WC claim is being contested (appealed).

2. A denial of Medicare benefits pending the outcome of the appeal would mean that the beneficiary may have to advance his own funds to pay for expenses that will eventually be paid by either Medicare or WC.

When WC does pay the claim, Medicare can collect the conditional payment it made from the WC carrier. If Medicare paid primary benefits in error, the overpayment is collected from the WC carrier. If Medicare duplicates payment made by the WC carrier, the overpayment will be collected from the party who received the payment (the physician or the beneficiary).

In situations where WC-related services plus other services are provided, the physician should submit two separate claim forms: one for the WC-related services to be submitted to WC; the other for the non-WC-related services to be submitted to Medicare. Separating the services in this way should speed processing and payment. If you are being treated for a job-related illness or injury and for other problems unrelated to your job, you may want to verify that your doctor's office is separating the services and submitting claims appropriately.

DISABLED

Medicare law provides that Medicare is the secondary payer for individuals who are entitled to Medicare based on disability and who also have coverage under a large group health plan.

Definitions

Large Group Health Plan (LGHP): Any health plan provided by or contributed to by an employer or an employee organization (including a self-insured plan) that provides health care directly or through insurance or reimbursement to employees or former employees, the employer, others associated or formerly associated with the employer in a business relationship, or their families; covers companies/organizations that normally employed at least 100 full- or part-time employees on a typical business day during the previous calendar year.

If the plan is a multi-employer plan, such as a union plan, which covers employees of some small employers and also employees of at least one employer that meets the 100 or more employees requirement, Medicare is secondary for all employees enrolled in the plan including those that work for small employers.

Employee: One who is actively working for an employer or, since disabled persons are not usually working, a person whose relationship to an employer indicates employee status. An individual who is not actively working may be considered an employee if:

- The individual is receiving payments from an employer that are subject to Federal Insurance Contributions Act (FICA) taxes (or would be subject to taxes except that the employer is not required to pay such taxes).

- The individual is termed an employee under state or federal law or in accordance with a court decision.

- The employer pays the same taxes for the individual as are paid for actively working employees.

- The individual continues to accrue vacation time or receives vacation pay.

- The individual participates in the employer's benefit plan, in which only employees may participate.

- The individual has rights to return to duty if the disabling condition improves.

- The individual continues to accrue sick leave.

To Whom the Provision Applies

Medicare is secondary to a LGHP for individuals who have LGHP coverage as a result of their own or a family member's current employment status. The disabled provision does not apply to:

- Individuals entitled, or who would be entitled upon application, to Medicare under the ESRD provision.

- Individuals who are covered by an EGHP of employer(s) of fewer than 100 employees, unless the EGHP is a multi-employer plan in which there is at least one employer of 100 or more employees.

- Individuals whose coverage by a LGHP is not based on either employment or a relationship to an employee, employer, or an individual associated with an employer in a business relationship.

Conditional Primary Payments

Medicare may pay conditional primary benefits in two situations:

1. The beneficiary has appealed or is protesting the LGHP denial of the claim (unless the LGHP offers only secondary coverage of services covered by Medicare).

2. The LGHP denied the claim because the time limit for filing the claim with the LGHP had expired (whether appealed or not).

Before making a conditional payment, Medicare will inform the beneficiary that both he and the LGHP insurer are responsible for reimbursing the Medicare program up to the amount it pays if the LGHP later pays the claim. The LGHP is responsible for reimbursing Medicare for the amount of the conditional benefits (up to the LGHP primary payment) if the LGHP pays primary benefits to the beneficiary. If the physician accepted assignment, Medicare will recover the excess Medicare payment from the party that received the LGHP payment. For unassigned claims, recovery will be attempted from the beneficiary.

END STAGE RENAL DISEASE

Medicare provides coverage to persons under age 65 who have ESRD. However, Medicare becomes a secondary payer for these individuals if they are also entitled to benefits through an EGHP. This provision went into effect on October 1, 1981. For dates of service on or after January 21, 1988, physicians and beneficiaries must first bill the EGHP. If the EGHP does not pay for covered services in full, Medicare may pay secondary benefits.

Also, the provision applies to all Medicare covered items and services, not just treatment of ESRD, furnished to beneficiaries who are in the waiting period.

Definitions

Employer: Individuals and organizations engaged in a trade or business and organizations exempt from income tax, such as religious, charitable, and educational institutions as well as the governments of the United States, the individual states, the District of Columbia, territories, Puerto Rico, Guam, and the Virgin Islands, including their agencies, instrumentalities, and political subdivisions. For purposes of the ESRD provision, employer is defined without regard to the number of employees.

Coordination Period: Refers to a period of up to 18 months during which Medicare benefits are secondary to benefits payable under an EGHP.

To Whom the Provision Applies

This provision applies to anyone entitled to Medicare solely on the basis of ESRD who also has coverage through an EGHP. It does not apply to beneficiaries entitled to Medicare because of age or disability.

Coordination Period

Prior to the enactment of the Omnibus Budget Reconciliation Act of 1990, the coordination period was 12 months. The legislation extended the coordination period to 18 months for beneficiaries who became eligible for or entitled to Medicare on or after February 1, 1990, and who began dialysis on or after December 1, 1989. Thus, beneficiaries whose 12-month coordination period ended on or before October 31, 1990, are not affected by this change; their coordination period remains at 12 months. This provision remains effective until September 30, 1998.

Medicare is the secondary payer to an EGHP for items and services beginning with the month in which a regular course of renal dialysis is initiated or, in the case of an individual who receives a kidney transplant, the first month in which the individual became entitled to Medicare. After the termination of the coordination period, Medicare becomes the primary payer.

Note that because ESRD beneficiaries have a three-month waiting period, the coordination period could actually be 21 months. The ESRD provision terminates with:

- The end of the coordination period.

- The first day of the month in which the beneficiary reaches age 65.

- The day the Medicare beneficiary is terminated from the EGHP.

- The beneficiary's date of death.

The coordination period is the most important—and most confusing—aspect of the ESRD secondary payer provision. Think of it simply: Medicare pays secondary benefits to an employer plan for a patient who is entitled to Medicare solely on the basis of ESRD for a period of 18 months. At the end of the 18-month coordination period (and the three-month waiting period), Medicare becomes the primary payer.

Conditional Primary Payments

Medicare may pay conditional primary benefits in two situations:

1. The beneficiary has appealed or is protesting the EGHP denial of the claim (unless the EGHP offers only secondary coverage of services covered by Medicare).

2. The EGHP denied the claim because the time limit for filing the claim with the EGHP had expired (whether appealed or not).

Before making a conditional payment, Medicare will inform the beneficiary that both he and the EGHP insurer are responsible for reimbursing the Medicare program up to the amount it pays if the EGHP later pays the claim. The EGHP is responsible for reimbursing Medicare for the amount of the conditional benefits (up to the EGHP primary payment) if the EGHP pays primary benefits to the beneficiary.

If the physician accepted assignment, Medicare will recover the excess Medicare payment from the party that received the EGHP payment. For unassigned claims, recovery will be attempted from the beneficiary.

Conditional Medicare benefits are not payable where an EGHP denies payment for particular services on the grounds that they are not covered by the plan but the Medicare carrier has reason to believe that the plan *does* cover the services. Also, conditional benefits are not payable if the EGHP offers only secondary coverage of services covered by Medicare, even if the EGHP has collected premiums only for secondary rather than primary coverage. The EGHP is obligated to pay primary benefits under the law; Medicare will not pay until the EGHP has made a determination on the claim.

AUTOMOBILE MEDICAL AND NO-FAULT

Under this provision, Medicare will not make payment for otherwise covered services to the extent that payment has been made, or can reasonably be expected to be made promptly, by any type of no-fault insurance. Effective for injuries occurring on or after December 5, 1980, this provision prohibits primary Medicare payment for treatment of injuries related to an accident when no-fault insurance could pay benefits.

This provision applies to services covered under automobile medical and no-fault insurance furnished on or after June 6, 1983, and to services covered under nonautomobile medical and no-fault insurance furnished on or after November 13, 1989. Medicare is secondary to no-fault insurance even if state law or a private insurance contract stipulates that benefits are secondary to Medicare benefits or otherwise limits its payments to Medicare beneficiaries.

Claims should be submitted to the no-fault insurer first. A claim for secondary benefits can be submitted if the no-fault insurer does not pay all of the charges on the claim. Medicare can pay for services related to an accident only if benefits are not currently available under the individual's no-fault insurance coverage because that insurance has paid maximum benefits for the accident.

Primary benefits cannot be paid by Medicare merely because the beneficiary wants to save insurance benefits to pay for future services or noncovered medical or nonmedical services. Primary benefits must be claimed to the no-fault insurer.

The no-fault provision terminates with the occurrence of one of the following:

- The date the case is settled with the no-fault insurer.

- The beneficiary's date of death.

Definitions

Automobile: Any self-propelled land vehicle of a type that must be registered and licensed in the state in which it is owned.

No-Fault Insurance: Insurance that pays for medical expenses for injuries sustained on the property or premises of the insured, or in the use, occupancy, or operation of an automobile, regardless of who may have been responsible for causing the accident. Examples of no-fault insurance include automobile no-fault insurance, often referred to as personal injury protection, and homeowners and commercial medical payments insurance, commonly referred to as Medpay coverage.

Liability Insurance: Insurance (including a self-insured plan) that provides payment based on legal liability for injuries, illness, or damages to property. It includes, but is not limited to, automobile liability, underinsured motorist, uninsured motorist, homeowners liability, malpractice, product liability, and general casualty insurance.

Underinsured Motorist Insurance: Insurance under which the policy holder's level of protection against losses caused by another is extended to compensate for inadequate coverage in the other party's policy or plan.

Uninsured Motorist Insurance: Liability insurance under which the policy holder's insurer pays for damages caused by a motorist who has no automobile liability insurance, carries less than the amount of insurance required by law, or is underinsured.

To Whom the Provision Applies

This provision applies to Medicare beneficiaries who are involved in an automobile or other type of accident. For example, Mr. Thomas is a 71-year-old Medicare beneficiary who sustains injuries in a car accident. For services related to treatment of the injuries sustained as a result of the accident, Mr. Thomas' automobile insurer is the primary payer. Medicare continues to pay primary benefits for services unrelated to the treatment of the injuries sustained in the accident.

Conditional Primary Benefits

In no-fault cases, conditional Medicare primary payments may be made under the following circumstances:

1. The beneficiary has filed a claim with the no-fault insurer and Medicare determines that the insurer will not pay promptly (within 120 days of receipt of the claim). Conditional payments are not made if the payment delay is due to the no-fault insurer claims that its benefits are secondary to Medicare.

2. The beneficiary, because of physical or mental incapacity, failed to meet a claim filing requirement of the no-fault insurer.

Conditional Medicare payments are made with the understanding that the beneficiary will reimburse the program to the extent that payment is subsequently made by the no-fault insurer.

LIABILITY

Liability insurance is insurance that pays for injuries sustained on someone's property. All companies have liability insurance that will pay medical bills related to an injury sustained on the company's property. For example, Mr. Jones falls in the grocery store parking lot and breaks his ankle. The grocery store's liability insurance is responsible for paying for treatment related to the broken ankle.

Effective for injuries sustained on or after December 5, 1980, Medicare is the secondary payer in situations where payment has been made, or can reasonably be expected to be made promptly, under a liability insurance plan/policy.

This provision terminates with the settlement of the liability case or with the death of the beneficiary.

Definitions

Self-Insured Plan: A plan under which an individual or other entity is authorized by state law to carry its own risk instead of taking out insurance with a carrier.

Accident: Any occurrence or activity that the individual believes resulted in injury or illness for which he holds another party liable.

To Whom the Provision Applies

This provision applies to Medicare beneficiaries who have been injured and are suing a person or other entity. The beneficiary typically is attempting to prove that the entity was negligent and that the negligence caused him to be injured. Medicare is the secondary payer for services related to any treatment of the injuries for which a liability insurer could be responsible for payment.

Conditional Primary Benefits

In the case of liability insurance, as contrasted to the other MSP categories, Medicare pays conditional primary benefits and then recovers when the liability insurer settles or pays. This is done because most liability cases take a long time to negotiate and settle; payment is not made promptly. Because of this, Medicare pays conditional benefits, monitors the case until it is resolved, and then recovers the conditional payment from the appropriate party.

PEER REVIEW ORGANIZATIONS BY STATE

ALABAMA
Alabama Quality
  Assurance Fdn., Inc.
Suite 200 North
One Perimeter Park South
Birmingham, AL
  35243-2327
(800) 760-3540

ALASKA
PRO-WEST
Suite 100
10700 Meridian Avenue,
  North
Seattle, WA 98133-9075
(800) 445-6941
(in Anchorage,
  dial 562-2252)

AMERICAN SAMOA
Hawaii Medical Service
  Association
818 Keeaumoku Street
P.O. Box 860
Honolulu, HI 96808-0860
(808) 944-3581 (will
  accept collect calls
  from out-of-state)

ARIZONA
Health Services Advisory
  Group, Inc.
301 East Bethany Home
  Road, B-157
Phoenix, AZ 85012
(800) 626-1577
[(800) 359-9909 or
  (800) 223-6693 in AZ]

ARKANSAS
Arkansas Foundation for
  Medical Care, Inc.
P.O. Box 2424
809 Garrison Avenue
Fort Smith, AR 72902
(800) 824-7586
[(800) 272-5528 in AR]

CALIFORNIA
California Medical
  Review, Inc.
Suite 500
60 Spear Street
San Francisco, CA 94105
(800) 841-1602 (in-state)
(415) 882-5800 (collect
  out-of-state calls OK)

COLORADO
Colorado Foundation for
  Medical Care
2821 South Parker Road
Aurora, CO 88014
(800) 727-7086 (in-state)
(303) 695-3333 (will
  accept collect calls from
  out-of-state)

CONNECTICUT
Connecticut Peer Review
  Organization, Inc.
Suite 200
100 Roscommon Drive
Middletown, CT 06457
(800) 553-7590 (in-state)
(203) 632-2008 (will
  accept collect calls from
  out-of-state)

DELAWARE
West Virginia Medical
  Institute, Inc.
3001 Chesterfield Place
Charleston, WV 25304
(800) 642-8686, ext. 266
(655-3077 in Wilmington)

DISTRICT OF
  COLUMBIA
Delmarva Foundation for
  Medical Care, Inc.
9240 Centreville Road
Easton, MD 21601
(800) 645-0011
[(800) 492-5811 in MD]

FLORIDA
Florida Medical Quality
  Assurance, Inc.
Suite 700
1211 N. Westshore Blvd.
Tampa, FL 33607
(800) 844-0795
(813) 281-9024

GEORGIA
Georgia Medical Care
  Foundation
Suite 200
57 Executive Park South
Atlanta, GA 30329
(800) 282-2614 (in-state)
(404) 982-0411

GUAM
Hawaii Medical Service
  Association
818 Keeaumoku Street
P.O. Box 860
Honolulu, HI 96808-0860
(808) 944-3581 (will
  accept collect calls from
  out-of-state)

HAWAII
Hawaii Medical Service
  Association
818 Keeaumoku Street
P.O. Box 860
Honolulu, HI 96808-0860
(808) 944-3581 (will
  accept collect calls from
  out-of-state)

IDAHO
PRO-WEST
Suite 100
10700 Meridian Avenue,
  North
Seattle, WA 98133-9075
(800) 445-6941
(208) 343-4617 (local
  Boise and collect)

ILLINOIS
Crescent Counties
  Foundation for
  Medical Care
1001 Warrenville Road
Lisle, IL 60532
(800) 647-8089
(708) 769-9600

INDIANA
Indiana Medical Review
  Organization
2901 Ohio Boulevard
P.O. Box 3713
Terre Haute, IN 47803
(800) 288-1499

IOWA
Iowa Foundation for
  Medical Care
Suite 350E
6000 Westown Parkway
West Des Moines, IA
  50266-7771
(800) 752-7014
(515) 223-2900

KANSAS
The Kansas Foundation
  for Medical Care, Inc.
2947 S.W. Wanamaker Dr
Topeka, KS 66614
(800) 432-0407 (in-state)
(913) 273-2552

KENTUCKY
Kentucky Medical Review
  Organization
10503 Timberwood
  Circle, Suite 200
P.O. Box 23540
Louisville, KY 40223
(800) 288-1499

LOUISIANA
Louisiana Health Care
  Review, Inc.
Suite 270
8591 United Plaza
  Boulevard
Baton Rouge, LA 70809
(800) 433-4958 (in-state)
(504) 926-6353

MAINE
Health Care Review, Inc.
Henry C. Hall Building
345 Blackstone Boulevard
Providence, RI 02906
(800) 541-9888 or
(800) 528-0700 (in-state)
(207) 945-0244 (will
  accept collect calls from
  out-of-state)

MARYLAND
Delmarva Foundation for
  Medical Care, Inc.
9240 Centreville Road
Easton, MD 21601
(800) 645-0011
[(800) 492-5811 in MD]

MASSACHUSETTS
Massachusetts Peer
  Review Organization
235 Wyman Street
Waltham, MA
  02154-1231
(800) 252-5533 (in-state)
(617) 890-0011 (will
  accept collect calls from
  out-of-state)

MICHIGAN
Michigan Peer Review
  Organization
Suite 200
40600 Ann Arbor Road
Plymouth, MI 48170-4495
(800) 365-5899

MINNESOTA
Foundation for Health
  Care Evaluation
Suite 400
2909 Metro Drive
Bloomington, MN 55425
(800) 444-3423

MISSISSIPPI
Mississippi Foundation
for Medical Care, Inc.
P.O. Box 4665
735 Riverside Drive
Jackson, MS 39296-4665
(800) 844-0600 (in-state)
(601) 948-8894

MISSOURI
Missouri Patient Care
Review Foundation
Suite 100
505 Hobbs Road
Jefferson City, MO 65109
(800) 347-1016

MONTANA
Montana-Wyoming
Foundation for
Medical Care
400 North Park,
Second Floor
Helena, MT 59601
(800) 497-8232 (in-state)
(406) 443-4020 (will
accept collect calls from
out-of-state)

NEBRASKA
Iowa Foundation for
Medical Care/The
Sunderbruch Corp.
Suite 350E
6000 Westown Parkway
West Des Moines, IA
50266
(800) 247-3004 (in-state)
(800) 422-4812

NEVADA
Nevada Peer Review
Suite 270
675 East 2100 South
Salt Lake City, UT
84106-1864
(800) 558-0829 (in NV)
(702) 826-1996 (in Reno)
(702) 835-9933 (will
accept collect calls from
out-of-state)

NEW HAMPSHIRE
New Hampshire Fdn.
for Medical Care
Suite 302
15 Old Rollinsford Road
Dover, NH 03820
(800) 582-7174 (in-state)
(603) 749-1641 (will
accept collect calls from
out-of-state)

NEW JERSEY
The Peer Review
  Organization of NJ
Central Division
Brier Hill Court,
  Building J
E. Brunswick, NJ 08816
(800) 624-4557 (in-state)
(908) 238-5570 (will
  accept collect calls from
  out-of-state)

NEW MEXICO
New Mexico Medical
  Review Association
707 Broadway N.E.,
  Suite 200
P.O. Box 27449
Albuquerque, NM
  87125-7449
(800) 279-6824 (in-state)
(505) 842-6326
(842-6236/Albuquerque)

NEW YORK
Island Peer Review
  Organization, Inc.
1979 Marcus Avenue,
  First Floor
Lake Success, NY 11042
(800) 331-7767 (in-state)
(516) 326-7767 (will
  accept collect calls from
  out-of-state)

NORTH CAROLINA
Medical Review of North
  Carolina
Suite 203
5625 Dillard Drive
P.O. Box 37309
Cary, NC 27511-9227
(800) 682-2650 (in-state)
(919) 851-2955

NORTH DAKOTA
North Dakota Health Care
  Review, Inc.
Suite 301
900 North Broadway
Minot, ND 58701
(800) 472-2902 (in-state)
(701) 852-4231 (will
  accept collect calls from
  out-of-state)

OHIO
Peer Review Systems
P.O. Box 6174
757 Brooksedge Plaza
  Drive
Westerville, OH
  43081-6174
(800) 837-0664
(800) 589-7337 (in-state)

OKLAHOMA
Oklahoma Foundation for
  Peer Review, Inc.
Suite 400, The Paragon
  Building
5801 Broadway Extension
Oklahoma City, OK
  73118-7489
(800) 522-3414 (in-state)
(405) 840-2891

PENNSYLVANIA
Keystone Peer Review
  Organization, Inc.
777 East Park Drive
P.O. Box 8310
Harrisburg, PA
  17105-8310
(800) 322-1914 (in-state)
(717) 564-8288

PUERTO RICO
Puerto Rico Foundation
  for Medical Care
Suite 605, Mercantile
  Plaza
Hato Rey, PR 00918
(809) 753-6705 (will
  accept collect calls from
  out-of-state)
(809) 753-6708 (will
  accept collect calls from
  out-of-state)

RHODE ISLAND
Health Care Review, Inc.
Henry C. Hall Building
345 Blackstone Boulevard
Providence, RI 02906
(800) 221-1691 (Region)
(800) 662-5028 (in-state)
(401) 331-6661 (will
  accept collect calls from
  out-of-state)

SOUTH CAROLINA
Medical Review of NC
Suite 203
5625 Dillard Drive
P.O. Box 37309
Cary, NC 27511-9227
(800) 682-2650 (in-state)
(919) 851-2955

SOUTH DAKOTA
South Dakota Foundation
  for Medical Care
1323 South Minnesota Av
Sioux Falls, SD 57105
(800) 658-2285

TENNESSEE
Mid-South Foundation for
  Medical Care
Suite 400
6401 Poplar Avenue
Memphis, TN 38119
(800) 489-4633

TEXAS
Texas Medical Foundation
Barton Oaks Plaza Two,
  Suite 200
901 Mopac Expressway
  South
Austin, TX 78746
(800) 725-8315 (in-state)
(512) 329-6610

UTAH
Utah Peer Review
  Organization
Suite 270
675 East 2100 South
Salt Lake City, UT
  84106-1864
(800) 274-2290

VERMONT
New Hampshire
  Foundation for Medical
  Care
Suite 302
15 Old Rollinsford Road
Dover, NH 03820
(800) 772-0151 (in-state)
(802) 655-6302 (will
  accept collect calls from
  out-of-state)

VIRGIN ISLANDS
Virgin Islands Medical
  Institute, Inc.
IAD Estate Diamond
  Ruby
P.O. Box 1566
Christiansted
St. Croix, U.S., VI
  00821-1566
(809) 778-6470 (will
  accept collect calls from
  out-of-state)

VIRGINIA
Medical Society of
  Virginia Review
  Organization
Suite 200
1606 Santa Rosa Road
P.O. Box K 70
Richmond, VA 23288
(800) 545-3814 (DC, MD
  and VA)
(804) 289-5320
(289-5397 in Richmond)

WASHINGTON
PRO-WEST
Suite 100
10700 Meridian Avenue,
  North
Seattle, WA 98133-9075
(800) 445-6941
(368-8272 in Seattle)

WEST VIRGINIA
West Virginia Medical
  Institute, Inc.
3001 Chesterfield Place
Charleston, WV 25304
(800) 642-8686, ext. 266
(346-9864 in Charleston)

WISCONSIN
Wisconsin Peer Review
  Organization
2909 Landmark Place
Madison, WI 53713
(800) 362-2320 (in-state)
(608) 274-1940

WYOMING
Montana-Wyoming
  Foundation for
  Medical Care
400 North Park,
  Second Floor
Helena, MT 59601
(800) 497-8232 (in-state)
(406) 443-4020 (will
  accept collect calls from
  out-of-state)

APPENDIX B

PART B CARRIER AND DMERC LISTING

The following is a list of all Medicare Part B carriers, and the four regional durable medical equipment carriers (DMERCs). The toll-free (800) numbers listed can typically only be used in the states where the carriers are located. Also listed are the local numbers which out-of-state callers may use. These numbers are for beneficiary use and should not be used by physicians, suppliers, or hospitals.

Part B Medicare Carriers

ALABAMA
Blue Cross and Blue
  Shield of Alabama
450 Riverchase Pkwy, E.
P.O. Box 830140
Birmingham, AL 35298
(205) 988–2244
(800) 292-8855

ALASKA
Aetna Life Insurance Co.
200 SW Market St.
P.O. Box 1998
Portland, OR 97207
(503) 222-6831
(800) 452-0125

AMERICAN SAMOA
Hawaii Medical Services
  Association
P.O. Box 860
Honolulu, HI 96808
(808) 944-2247

ARIZONA
Aetna Life Insurance Co.
P.O. Box 37200
Phoenix, AZ 85069
(602) 861-1968
(800) 352-0411

ARKANSAS
Arkansas Blue Cross and
  Blue Shield
601 Gaines St.
P.O. Box 1418
Little Rock, AR 72203
(501) 378–2320
(800) 482-5525

CALIFORNIA
For Los Angeles, Orange,
San Diego, Ventura,
Imperial, San Luis
Obispo, and Santa
Barbara counties:
Transamerica Occidental
  Life Insurance Co.
Box 30540
Los Angeles, CA 90030
(213) 748-2311
(800) 675-2266

For rest of state:
Medicare Claims
  Department
Blue Shield of California
Chico, CA 95976
For area codes 209, 408,
415, 510, 707, and 916:
(916) 743-1583
(800) 952-8627

CALIFORNIA (cont.)
For area codes 213, 310,
619, 714, 805, 818, and
909:
(714) 796-9393
(800) 848-7713

COLORADO
Blue Shield of Colorado
Governor's Center II
600 Grant Street
Suite 600
Denver, CO 80203
(701) 282-0691
(800) 247-2267

CONNECTICUT
The Travelers Insurance
  Company
538 Preston Avenue
P.O. Box 9000
Meriden, CT 06454
(203) 728-6783 (Hartford)
(203) 237-8592 (Meriden)
(800) 982-6819

DELAWARE
Xact Medicare Services
P.O. Box 890065
Camp Hill, PA 17089
(800) 233-1124

DISTRICT OF COLUMBIA

Xact Medicare Services
P.O. Box 890065
Camp Hill, PA 17089
(800) 233-1124

FLORIDA

Blue Cross and Blue
  Shield of Florida, Inc.
532 Riverside Avenue
17th and 18th Floors
P.O. Box 2360
Jacksonville, FL 32231
*For copies of EOMB
notices, requests for
MEDPARD directories,
brief claims inquiries
(status or verification of
receipt), and address
changes, call:*
(904) 355-8899
(800) 666-7586

*For all other Medicare
needs, call:*
(904) 355-3680
(800) 333-7586

GEORGIA

Aetna Life Insurance
  Company
P.O. Box 3018
Savannah, GA 31402
(912) 920-2412
(800) 727-0827

GUAM

Aetna Life Insurance
  Company
P.O. Box 3947
Honolulu, HI 96812
(808) 524-1240

HAWAII

Aetna Life Insurance
  Company
P.O. Box 3947
Honolulu, HI 96812
(808) 524-1240
(800) 272-5242

IDAHO

CIGNA Medicare
3150 N. Lakeharbor Lane,
  Suite 254
P.O. Box 8048
Boise, ID 83707
(208) 342-7763
(800) 627-2782

ILLINOIS
Medicare Claims/Health
  Care Service Corp.
P.O. Box 4422
Marion, IL 62959
(317) 842-4151
(800) 642-6930

INDIANA
Medicare AdminaStar
  Federal
P.O. Box 7073
Indianapolis, IN 46207
(317) 842-4151
(800) 622-4792

IOWA
IASD Health Services
  Corporation
dba Blue Cross and Blue
  Shield of Iowa

Correspondence:
P.O. Box 9269
Des Moines, IA 50306

Claims:
P.O. Box 10491
Des Moines, IA 50360
(515) 245-4785
(800) 532-1285

KANSAS
*For Johnson and Wyan-
dotte counties:*
Blue Cross and Blue
  Shield of Kansas, Inc.
P.O. Box 419840
Kansas City, MO 64141
(816) 561-0900
(800) 892-5900

For rest of state:
Blue Cross and Blue
  Shield of Kansas, Inc.
1133 S.W. Topeka Blvd.
P.O. Box 239
Topeka, KS 66629
(913) 232-3773
(800) 432-3531

KENTUCKY
AdminaStar of Kentucky
P.O. Box 37630
Louisville, KY 50233
(502) 425-6759
(800) 999-7608

LOUISIANA
Blue Cross and Blue
  Shield of Louisiana
Medicare Administration
P.O. Box 98501
Baton Rouge, LA 70884
(504) 529-1494 (New
  Orleans)
(504) 927-3490 (Baton
  Rouge)
(800) 462-9666

MAINE
C and S Administrative
  Services
P.O. Box 1000
Hingham, MA 02044
(207) 828-4300
(800) 492-0919

MARYLAND
*For Montgomery and
Prince Georges counties:*
Xact Medicare Services
P.O. Box 890065
Camp Hill, PA 17089
(800) 233-1124

For rest of state:
Trail Blazer Enterprises
P.O. Box 5678
Timonium, MD 21094
(800) 492-4795

MASSACHUSETTS
C and S Administrative
  Services
P.O. Box 1000
Hingham, MA 02044
(617) 741-3300
(800) 882-1228

MICHIGAN
Healthcare Services
  Corporation
Michigan Medicare
  Claims
P.O. Box 5544
Marion, IL 62959
(313) 225-8200
(800) 482-4045

MINNESOTA
*For Anoka, Dakota, Fill-
more, Goodhue, Henne-
pin, Houston, Olmstead,
Ramsey, Wabasha, Wash-
ington, and Winona
counties:*
The Travelers Insurance
  Company
8120 Penn Avenue South
Bloomington, MN 55431
(612) 884-7171
(800) 352-2762

MINNESOTA (cont.)
For rest of state:
Blue Cross and Blue
  Shield of Minnesota
P.O. Box 64357
St. Paul, MN 55164
(612) 456-5070
(800) 392-0343

MISSISSIPPI
The Travelers Insurance
  Company
P.O. Box 22545
Jackson, MS 39225
(601) 956-0372
(800) 682-5417

MISSOURI
*For Andrew, Atchison,
Bates, Benton, Buchanan,
Caldwell, Carroll, Cass,
Clay, Clinton, Daviess,
DeKalb, Gentry, Grundy,
Harrison, Henry, Holt,
Jackson, Johnson,
Lafayette, Livingston,
Mercer, Nodaway, Pettis,
Platte, Ray, St. Clair,
Saline, Vernon, and
Worth counties:*

MISSOURI (cont.)
Blue Cross and Blue
  Shield of Kansas, Inc.
P.O. Box 419840
Kansas City, MO 64141
(816) 561-0900
(800) 392-3070

For rest of state:
General American Life
  Insurance Company
P.O. Box 505
St. Louis, MO 63166
(314) 843-8880
(800) 392-3070

MONTANA
Blue Cross and Blue
  Shield of Montana, Inc.
2501 Beltview
P.O. Box 4310
Helena, MT 59604
(406) 444-8350
(800) 332-6146

NEBRASKA
Blue Cross and Blue
  Shield of Kansas, Inc.
P.O. Box 419840
Kansas City, MO 64141
(816) 561-0900
(800) 392-3070

NEBRASKA (cont.)

Claims should be sent to:
Blue Cross and Blue
  Shield of Nebraska
P.O. Box 3106
Omaha, NB 68103
(800) 633-1113

NEVADA

Aetna Life Insurance
  Company
P.O. Box 37230
Phoenix, AZ 85069
(602) 861-1968
(800) 528-0311

NEW HAMPSHIRE

C and S Administrative
  Services
P.O. Box 1000
Hingham, MA 02044
(207) 828-4300
(800) 447-1142

NEW JERSEY

Xact Medicare Services
P.O. Box 890065
Camp Hill, PA 17089
(800) 462-9306

NEW MEXICO

Aetna Life Insurance
  Company
P.O. Box 25500
Oklahoma City, OK
  73125
(505) 821-3350
(800) 423-2925

NEW YORK

*For Bronx, Columbia,
Delaware, Dutchess,
Greene, Kings, Nassau,
New York, Orange, Put-
nam, Richmond, Rock-
land, Suffolk, Sullivan,
Ulster, and Westchester
counties:*
Empire Blue Cross and
  Blue Shield
P.O. Box 2280
Peekskill, NY 10566
(516) 244-5100
(800) 442-8430

For Queens County:
Group Health, Inc.
P.O. Box 1608
Ansonia Station
New York, NY 10023
(212) 721-1770

NEW YORK (cont.)

For rest of state:
Blue Cross and Blue
  Shield of Western
  New York
Upstate Medicare Div.
33 Lewis
Binghamton, NY 13905
(800) 252-6550

NORTH CAROLINA

Connecticut General Life
  Insurance Company
P.O. Box 671
Nashville, TN 37202
(919) 665-0348
(800) 672-3071

NORTH DAKOTA

Blue Shield of North
  Dakota
711 Second Avenue, N.
Fargo, ND 58102
(701) 277-2363
(800) 247-2267

NORTHERN
 MARIANA ISLANDS

Aetna Life Insurance
P.O. Box 3947
Honolulu, HI 96812
(808) 524-1240

OHIO

Nationwide Mutual
  Insurance Co.
P.O. Box 57
Columbus, OH 43216
(614) 249-7157
(800) 522-9079

OKLAHOMA

Aetna Life Insurance
701 N.W. 63rd Street
Oklahoma City, OK
  73116
(405) 848-7711
(800) 522-9079

OREGON

Aetna Life Insurance
P.O. Box 1997
Portland, OR 97207
(503) 222-6831
(800) 452-0125

PENNSYLVANIA

*For Philadelphia, Bucks,
Montgomery, Chester and
Delaware counties:*
Veritus, Inc.
dba Blue Cross of
  Western Pennsylvania
Fifth Avenue Place
120 Fifth Avenue
Pitsburgh, PA 15222
(412) 255-7000

PENNSYLVANIA (cont.)
For rest of state:
Xact Medicare Services
Box 890065
Camp Hill, PA 17089
(800) 382-1274

PUERTO RICO
Triple-S, Inc.
P.O. Box 71391
San Juan, PR 00936
(809) 749-4900
(800) 981-7015

RHODE ISLAND
Blue Cross and Blue
  Shield of Rhode Island
444 Westminster Street
Providence, RI 02903
(401) 861-2273
(800) 662-5170

SOUTH CAROLINA
Blue Cross and Blue
  Shield of South Carolina
Medicare Operations
P.O. Box 100190
Columbia, SC 29202
(803) 788-3882
(800) 868-2522

SOUTH DAKOTA
Blue Shield of North
  Dakota
711 Second Avenue, N.
Fargo, ND 58102
(800) 437-4762

TENNESSEE
CIGNA Medicare
P.O. Box 1465
Nashville, TN 37202
(615) 244-5650
(800) 342-8900

TEXAS
Blue Cross and Blue
  Shield of Texas, Inc.
P.O. Box 660031
Dallas, TX 75266
(214) 235-3433
(800) 442-2620

UTAH
Blue Shield of Utah
P.O. Box 30269
Salt Lake City, UT 84130
(801) 481-6196
(800) 426-3477

VERMONT
C and S Administrative
  Services
P.O. Box 1000
Hingham, MA 02044
(207) 828-4300
(800) 447-1142

VIRGIN ISLANDS
Triple-S, Inc.
P.O. Box 71391
San Juan, PR 00936
(809) 774-7915 (St.
  Thomas)
(809) 773-9548 (St.
  Croix)
(800) 474-7448

VIRGINIA
*For Arlington and Fairfax
counties and cities of
Alexandria, Falls Church,
and Fairfax:*
Xact Medicare Services
P.O. Box 890065
Camp Hill, PA 17089
(800) 233-1124

For rest of state:
The Travelers Insurance
  Company
P.O. Box 26463
Richmond, VA 23261

VIRGINIA (cont.)
(804) 330-4786
(800) 552-3423

WASHINGTON
Aetna Life Insurance
P.O. Box 91099
Seattle, WA 98111
(206) 621-0359
(800) 372-6604

WEST VIRGINIA
Nationwide Mutual
  Insurance Company
P.O. Box 57
Columbus, OH 43216
(614) 249-7157
(800) 848-0106

WISCONSIN
Wisconsin Physicians'
  Service
Box 1787
Madison, WI 53701
(608) 221-3330
(800) 944-0051

WYOMING
Blue Cross and Blue
  Shield of North Dakota
P.O. Box 9379
Fargo, ND 58106
(307) 632-9381
(800) 442-2371

Durable Medical Equipment
Regional Carriers (DMERCs)

REGION A

For Connecticut, Delaware, Maine, Massachusetts, New Hampshire, New Jersey, New York, Pennsylvania, Rhode Island, Vermont:
MetraHealth Insurance
  Company
P.O. Box 6800
Wilks-Barre, PA 18773
(717) 735-9400
(800) 842-2052

REGION B

For District of Columbia, Illinois, Indiana, Maryland, Michigan, Ohio, Virginia, West Virginia, Wisconsin:
AdminaStar Federal, Inc.
P.O. Box 7027
Indianapolis, IN 46207
(317) 577-5722
(800) 952-2063

REGION C

For Alabama, Arkansas, Colorado, Florida, Georgia, Kentucky, Louisiana, Mississippi, New Mexico,

REGION C (cont.)

North Carolina, Oklahoma, Puerto Rico, South Carolina, Tennessee, Texas, Virgin Islands:
Palmetto Government
  Benefits
  Administrators
Medicare DMERC
  Operations
P.O. Box 100222
Columbia, SC 29202
(800) 213-5451

REGION D

For Alaska, Arizona, California, Guam, Hawaii, Idaho, Iowa, Kansas, Missouri, Montana, Nebraska, Nevada, North Dakota, Oregon, South Dakota, Utah, Washington, Wyoming:
CIGNA
Medicare Region D
  DMERC
P.O. Box 690
Nashville, TN 37202
(615) 244-5600

APPENDIX C

COVERED DURABLE MEDICAL EQUIPMENT (DME) ITEMS

Item	Coverage Status
Air Cleaners	Deny; Environmental control equipment, not primarily medical in nature (§1861(n) of the Act)
Air Conditioners	Deny; Environmental control equipment, not primarily medical in nature (§1861(n) of the Act)
Air-Fluidized Bed	See §60-19
Alternating Pressure Pads and Mattresses, and Lambs' Wool Pads	Covered if patient has, or is highly susceptible to, decubitus ulcers, and patient's physician has specified that he will be supervising its use in connection with his course of treatment
Audible/Visible Signal Monitor	See Self-Contained Pacemaker Monitor
Augmentative Communication Device	See Communicator
Bathtub Lifts	Deny; Convenience item, not primarily medical in nature (§1861(n) of the Act)
Bathtub Seats	Deny; Comfort or convenience item, hygienic equipment; not primarily medical in nature (§1861(n) of the Act)
Bead Bed	See §60-19

Item	Coverage Status
Bed Baths (home type)	Deny; Hygienic equipment, not primarily medical (§1861(n) of the Act)
Bed Lifter (bed elevator)	Deny; Not primarily medical in nature (§1861(n) of the Act)
Bedboards	Deny; Not primarily medical in nature (§1861(n) of the Act)
Bed Pans (autoclavable hosptial type)	Covered if patient is bed confined
Bed Side Rails	See Hospital Beds, §60-18
Beds-Lounge (power or manual	Deny; Not a hospital bed, comfort or convenience item, not primarily medical in nature (§1861(n) of the Act)
Beds-Oscillating	Deny; Institutional equipment, inappropriate for home use
Bidet Toilet Seat	See Toilet Seats
Blood Glucose Analyzer-Reflectance Colorimeter	Deny; Unsuitable for home use (See §60-11)
Blood Glucose Monitor	Covered if patient meets certain conditions (See §60-11)
Braille Teaching Texts	Deny; Educational equipment, not primarily medical in nature (§1861(n) of the Act)
Canes	Covered if patient's condition impairs ambulation (See §60-3)
Carafes	Deny; Convenience item, not primarily medical in nature (§1861(n) of the Act)

Item	Coverage Status
Catheters	Deny; Nonreusable disposable supply (§1861(n) of the Act)
Commodes	Covered if patient is confined to bed or room

NOTE: The term "room confined" means that the patient's condition is such that leaving the room is medically contraindicated. The accessibility of bathroom facilities generally would not be a factor in this determination. However, confinement of a patient to his home in a case where there are no toilet facilities in the home may be equated to room confinement. Moreover, payment may also be made if a patient's medical condition confines him to a floor of his home and there is no bathroom located on that floor.

Item	Coverage Status
Communicator	Deny; Convenience item, not primarily medical in nature (§1861(n) of the Act)
Continuous Passive Motion Device (CPM)	Covered for patients who have received a total knee replacement. To qualify for coverage, use of the device must commence within two days following surgery. In addition, coverage is limited to that portion of the three-week period following surgery during which the device is used in the patient's home

There is insufficient evidence to justify coverage of these devices for longer periods of time or for other applications.

Item	Coverage Status
Continuous Positive Airway Pressure (CPAP)	See §60-17
Crutches	Covered if patient's condition impairs ambulation

Item	Coverage Status
Cushion Lift Power Seat	See Seat Lifts
Dehumidifiers (room or central heating type)	Deny; Environmental control equipment primarily medical in nature (§1861(n) of the Act)
Diathermy Machines (standard and pulse wave types)	Deny; Inappropriate for home use (See §35-41)
Digital Electronic Pacemaker Monitor	See Self-Contained Pacemaker Monitor
Disposable Sheets Bags	Deny; Nonreusable disposable supplies and (§1861(n) of the Act)
Elastic Stockings	Deny; Nonreusable supply, not rental-type items
Electric Air Cleaners	Deny; See Air Cleaners (§1861(n) of the Act)
Electric Hospital Beds	See Hospital Beds (§60-18)
Electrostatic Machines	Deny; See Air Cleaners and Air Conditioners (§1861(n) of the Act)
Elevators	Deny; Convenience item, not primarily medical in nature (§1861(n) of the Act)
Emesis Basins	Deny; Convenience item, not primarily medical in nature (§1861(n) of the Act)
Esophageal Dilator	Deny; Physician instrument, inappropriate for patient use

Item	Coverage Status
Exercise Equipment	Deny; Not primarily medical in nature (§1861(n) of the Act)
Fabric Supports	Deny; Nonreusable supplies, not rental-type item (§1861(n) of the Act)
Face Masks (oxygen)	Covered if oxygen is covered (See §60-4)
Face Masks (surgical)	Deny; Nonreusable disposable items (§1861(n) of the Act)
Flowmeter	See Medical Oxygen Regulators
Fluidic Breathing Assister	See IPPB Machines
Fomentation Device	See Heating Pads
Gel Flotation Pads and Mattresses	See Alternating Pressure Pads and Mattresses
Grab Bars	Deny; Self-help device, not primarily medical in nature (§1861(n) of the Act)
Heat and Massage Foam Cushion Pad	Deny; Not primarily medical in nature, personal comfort item (§1861(n) of the Act)
Heating and Cooling Plants	Deny; Environmental control equipment not primarily medical in nature (§1861(n) of the Act)
Heating Pads	Covered if the contractor's medical staff determines patient's medical condition is one for which the application of heat in the form of a heating pad is therapeutically effective

Item	Coverage Status
Heat Lamps	Covered if the contractor's medical staff determines patient's medical condition is one for which the application of heat in the form of a heating pad is therapeutically effective
Hospital Beds	See §60-18
Hot Packs	See Heating Pads
Humidifiers (oxygen)	See Oxygen Humidifiers
Humidifiers (room or central heating types	Deny; Environmental control equipment not medical in nature (§1861(n) of Act)
Hydraulic Lift	See Patient Lifts
Incontinent Pads	Deny; Nonreusable supply, hygienic item (§1861(n) of the Act)
Infusion Pumps	For external and implantable pumps, see §60-14; If the pump is used with an enteral or parenteral nutritional therapy system, see 65-10 to 65-10.2 for special coverage rules
Injectors (hypodermic jet pressure-powered devices for injection of insulin)	Deny; Effectiveness not adequately demonstrated
IPPB Machines	Covered if patient's ability to breathe is severely impaired
Iron Lungs	See Ventilators
Irrigating Kit	Deny; Nonreusable supply, hygienic equipment (§1861(n) of the Act)

Appendix C: Covered Durable Medical Equipment (DME)

Item	Coverage Status
Lambs' Wool Pads	Covered under same conditions as alternating pressure pads/mattresses
Leotards	Deny; See Pressure Leotards (§1861(n) of the Act)
Lymphedema Pumps (segmental and non-segmental therapy types)	Covered, See §60-16
Massage Devices	Deny; Personal comfort items, not primarily medical in nature (§1861(n) and 1862(a)(6) of the Act)
Mattress	Covered only where hospital bed is medically necessary; Separate charge for replacement mattress should not be allowed where hospital bed with mattress is rented. See §60-18
Medical Oxygen Regulators	Covered only if patient's ability to breathe is severely impaired See §60-4
Mobile Geriatric Chair	See Rolling Chairs
Motorized Wheelchairs	See Wheelchairs (power operated)
Muscle Stimulators	Covered for certain conditions, See §35-77
Nebulizers	Covered if patient's ability to breathe is severely impaired
Oscillating Beds	Deny; Institutional equipment, inappropriate for home use
Overbed Tables	Deny; Convenience item, not primarily medical in nature (§1861(n) of the Act)

Item	Coverage Status
Oxygen	Covered if the oxygen has been prescribed for use in connection with medically necessary durable medical equipment (See §60-4)
Oxygen Humidifiers	Covered if a medical humidifier has been prescribed for use in connection with medically necessary durable medical equipment for purposes of moisturizing oxygen (See §60-4)
Oxygen Regulators	See Medical Oxygen Regulators (medical)
Oxygen Tents	See §60-4
Paraffin Bath Units (portable)	See Portable Paraffin Bath Units
Parrafin Bath Units (standard)	Deny; Institutional equipment, inappropriate for home use.
Parallel Bars	Deny; Support exercise equipment, primarily for institutional use; in the home setting other devices (e.g., a walker) satisy the patient's need
Patient Lifts	Covered if contractor's medical staff determines patient's condition is such that periodic movement is necessary to effect improvement or to arrest or retard deterioration in his condition

Item	Coverage Status
Percussors	Covered for mobilizing respiratory tract secretions in patients with chronic obstructive lung disease, chronic bronchitis, or emphysema, when patient or operator of powered percussor has received appropriate training by a physician or therapist, and no one competent to administer manual therapy is available

Portable Oxygen Systems:

Item	Coverage Status
Regulated (adjustable flow rate)	Covered under the conditions specified in §60-4; Refer all claims to medical staff for this determination
Preset (flow rate not adjustable)	Deny; Emergency, first-aid, or precautionary equipment, essentially not therapeutic in nature
Portable Paraffin Bath	Covered when the patient has undergone a successful trial period of paraffin therapy ordered by a physician and the patient's condition is expected to be relieved by long term use of this modality
Portable Room Heaters	Deny; Environmental control equipment, not primarily medical in nature (§1861(n) of the Act)
Portable Whirlpool Pumps	Deny; Personal comfort items, not primarily medical in nature (1862(a)(6) and §1861(n) of the Act)
Postural Drainage Boards	Covered if patient has a chronic pulmonary condition

Item	Coverage Status
Preset Portable Oxygen Units	Deny; Emergency, first-aid, or pre-cautionary equipment, essentially not therapeutic in nature
Pressure Leotards	Deny; Nonreusable supply, not rental-type item (§1861(n) of the Act)
Pulse Tachometer	Deny; Not reasonable or necessary for monitoring pulse of homebound patient with or without a cardiac pacemaker
Quad-Canes	See Walkers
Raised Toilet Seats	Deny; Convenience item, hygienic equipment, not primarily medical in nature (§1861(n) of the Act)
Reflectance Colorimeters	See Blood Glucose Analyzers
Respirators	See Ventilators
Rolling Chairs	Covered if the contractor's medical staff determines that the patient's condition is such that there is a medical need for this item and it has been prescribed by the patient's physician in lieu of a wheelchair. Coverage is limited to those rollabout chairs having casters of at least 5 inches in diameter and specifically designed to meet the needs of ill, injured, or otherwise impaired individuals.

Note: Coverage is denied for the wide range of chairs with smaller casters as are found in general use in homes, offices, and institutions for many purposes not related to the care or treatment of ill or injured persons. This type is not primarily medical in nature (§1861(n) of the Act).

Item	Coverage Status
Safety Roller	See §60-15
Sauna Baths	Deny; Not primarily medical in nature, personal comfort items (§1861(n) and 1862(a)(6) of the Act)
Seat Lift	Covered under the conditions specified in §60-8; Refer all to medical staff for this determination
Self-Contained Pacemaker Monitor	Covered when prescribed by a physician for a patient with a cardiac pacemaker (See 50-1C and §60-7)
Sitz Bath	Covered if the contractor's medical staff determines that the patient has an infection or injury in the perineal area and the item has been prescribed by the patient's physician as a part of his planned regimen of treatment in the patient's home
Spare Tanks of Oxygen	Deny; Convenience or precautionary supply
Speech Teaching Machine	Deny; Education equipment, not primarily medical in nature (§1861(n) of the Act)
Stairway Elevators	Deny; See Elevators
Standing Table	Deny; Convenience item, not primarily medical in nature (§1861(n) of the Act)
Steam Packs	These packs are covered under the same condition as a heating pad (See Heating Pads)

Item	Coverage Status
Suction Machine	Covered if the contractor's medical staff determines that the machine specified in the claim is medically required and appropriate for home use without technical or professional supervision
Support Hose	Deny; See Fabric Supports
Surgical Leggings	Deny; Nonreusable supply, not rental-type item (§1861(n) of the Act)
Telephone Alert Systems	Deny; These are emergency communication systems and do not serve a diagnostic or therapeutic purpose
Telephone Arms	Deny; Convenience item; not medical in nature (§1861(n) of the Act)
Toilet Seats	Deny; Not medical equipment (§1861(n) of the Act)
Traction Equipment	Covered if patient has orthopedic impairment requiring traction equipment which prevents ambulation during the period of use; Consider covering devices usable during ambulation, e.g., cervical traction collar, under the brace provision
Trapeze Bars	Covered if patient is bed confined and the patient needs a trapeze bar to sit up because of respiratory condition, to change body position for other medical reasons, or to get in and out of bed
Treadmill Exerciser	Deny; Exercise equipment, not primarily medical in nature (§1861(n) of the Act)

Item	Coverage Status
Ultraviolet Cabinet	Covered for selected patients with generalized intractable psoriasis; Using appropriate consultation, the contractor should determine whether medical and other factors justify treatment at home rather than at alternative sites, e.g., outpatient department of a hospital
Urinals (autoclavable hospital type)	Covered if patient is bed confined
Vaporizers	Covered if patient has a respiratory illness
Ventilators	Covered for treatment of neuromuscular diseases, thoracic restrictive diseases, and chronic respiratory failure consequent to chronic obstructive pulmonary disease; Includes both positive and negative pressure types
Walkers	Covered if patient's condition impairs ambulation; See also §60-15
Water and Pressure Pad/ Mattress	See Alternating Pressure Pads and Mattresses
Wheelchairs	Covered if patient's condition is such that without the use of a wheelchair he would otherwise be bed or chair confined; An individual may qualify for a wheelchair and still be considered bed confined

Item	Coverage Status
Wheelchairs (power) and Wheelchairs With Other features	Covered if patient's medical condition is such that a wheelchair is medically necessary and the patient is unable to operate the wheelchair manually; Any claim involving a power wheelchair or a wheelchair with other special features should be referred for medical consultation since payment for special features is limited to those which are medically required because of the patient's condition (See §60-5 for power operated and §60-6 for specially sized wheelchairs)

NOTE: A power operate vehicle that may appropriately be used as a wheelchair can be covered. See §60-5 for coverage details

Whirlpool Bath Equipment (standard)	Covered if patient is homebound and has a condition for which the whirlpool bath can be expected to provide substantial therapeutic benefit justifying its cost; Where the patient is not homebound but has such a condition, payment is restricted to the cost of providing the services elsewhere, e.g., an outpatient department of a participating hospital, if that alternative is less costly. In all cases, refer claim to medical staff for a determination
Whirlpool Pumps	Deny; See Portable Whirlpool Pumps
White Cane	Deny; See §60-3

APPENDIX D

STATE INSURANCE DEPARTMENTS AND AGENCIES ON AGING

Each state has its own laws and regulations governing all types of insurance. The insurance offices are responsible for enforcing those laws, as well as providing the public with information about insurance. Insurance counseling services are available by calling the number listed.

The agencies on aging are responsible for coordinating services for older persons.

ALABAMA
Insurance Department
Consumer Service
  Division
135 S. Union St.
P.O. Box 30351
Montgomery, AL 36130
(334) 269-3550

Insurance Counseling
(800) 243-5463

Commission on Aging
770 Washington Ave.
  Suite 470
P.O. Box 301851
Montgomery, AL 36130
(334) 242-5743

ALASKA
Division of Insurance
800 E. Dimond, Suite 560
Anchorage, AK 99515
(907) 349-1230

Insurance Counseling
(800) 478-6065
(907) 562-7249

**Older Alaskans
  Commission**
P.O. Box 110209
Juneau, AK 99811-0209
(907) 465-3250

AMERICAN SAMOA
Insurance Department
Office of the Governor
Pago Pago, AS 96799
011 (684) 633-4116

**Territorial Admini-
stration on Aging**
Gvmt of American Somoa
Pago Pago, AS 96799
011 (684) 633-1252

ARIZONA
Insurance Department
Consumer Affairs
  Division
2910 N. 44th St.
Phoenix, AZ 85018
(602) 912-8444

Insurance Counseling
(800) 432-4040
(602) 542-6595

Aging and Adult Adm.
Department of Economic
  Security
1789 W. Jefferson St.
Phoenix, AZ 85007
(602) 542-4446

ARKANSAS
Insurance Department
Seniors Insurance
  Network
1123 S. University Ave.
Suite 400
Little Rock, AR 72204
(800) 852-5494

Insurance Counseling
(800) 852-5494
(501) 686-2940

**Division of Aging and
  Adult Services**
1417 Donaghey Plaza S.
P.O. Box 1437/Slot 1412
Little Rock, AR
  72203-1437
(501) 682-2441

CALIFORNIA
Insurance Department
Consumer Services
  Division
300 S. Spring St.
Los Angeles, CA 90013
(213) 897-8921

Insurance Counseling
(800) 927-4357
(916) 323-7315

CALIFORNIA (cont.)
Department of Aging
1600 K St.
Sacramento, CA 95814
(916) 322-3887

COLORADO
Insurance Division
1560 Broadway
  Suite 850
Denver, CO 80202
(303) 894-7499, ext. 356

Insurance Counseling
(800) 544-9181

Aging and Adult
  Services
Dept of Social Services
1575 Sherman St., 4th Fl.
Denver, CO 80203-1714
(303) 866-3851

CONNECTICUT
Insurance Department
P.O. Box 816
Hartford, CT 06142-0816
(203) 297-3800

Insurance Counseling
(800) 443-9946

CONNECTICUT (cont.)
Elderly Services Division
175 Main St.
Hartford, CT 06106
(800) 443-9946

DELAWARE
Insurance Department
Rodney Building
841 Silver Lake Blvd.
Dover, DE 19904
(302) 739-4251
(800) 282-8611

Insurance Counseling
(800) 336-9500

Division of Aging
Department of Health and
  Social Services
1901 N. DuPont Highway
  2nd Fl. Annex
Administration Building
New Castle, DE 19720
(302) 577-4791

DISTRICT OF COLUMBIA
Insurance Department
Consumer and
  Professional Services
  Bureau
441 4th St., N.W.
  Suite 850 North
Washington, D.C. 20001
(202) 727-8000

Insurance Counseling
(202) 994-7463

Office on Aging
441 4th St. NW, 9th Fl.
Washington, DC 20001
(202) 724-5626
(202) 724-5622

FLORIDA
Insurance Department
200 E. Gaines St.
Tallahassee, FL 32399
(904) 922-3100

Insurance Counseling
(904) 922-2073

FLORIDA (cont.)
Department of Elder Affairs
1317 Winewood Blvd.
Building 1, Room 317
Tallahassee, FL
  32399-0700
(904) 922-5297

GEORGIA
Insurance Department
2 MLK Jr. Drive
716 West Tower
Atlanta, GA 30334
(404) 656-2056

Insurance Counseling.
(800) 669-8387

Division of Aging Svcs
Department of Human
  Resources
2 Peachtree St., NW,
  Room 18.403
Atlanta, GA 30303
(404) 657-5258

GUAM
Insurance Department
Department of Revenue
and Taxation
378 Chalan San Antonio
Tamuning, Guam 96911
011 (671) 477-5144

**Division of Senior
Citizens**
Department of Public
Health and Social
Services
P.O. Box 2816
Agana, Guam 96910
011 (617) 632-4141

HAWAII
Insurance Division
Department of Commerce
and Consumer Affairs
P.O. Box 3614
Honolulu, HI 96811
(808) 586-2790

Insurance Counseling
(808) 586-0100

**Executive Office on
Aging**
335 Merchant St.,
Room 241
Honolulu, HI 96813
(808) 586-0100

IDAHO
Insurance Department
SHIBA Program
700 W. State St.,
3rd Floor
Boise, ID 83720-0043
(208) 334-4350

Insurance Counseling
SW: (800) 247-4422
North: (800) 488-5725
SE: (800) 488-5764
Central: (800) 488-5731

Office on Aging
Statehouse, Room 108
Boise, ID 83720
(208) 334-3833

ILLINOIS
Insurance Department
320 W. Washington St.
4th Floor
Springfield, IL 62767
(217) 782-4515

Insurance Counseling
(800) 548-9034

Department on Aging
421 E. Capitol Ave.
Springfield, IL 62701
(217) 785-3356

INDIANA
Insurance Department
311 W. Washington St.
Suite 300
Indianapolis, IN 46204
(317) 232-2395

Insurance Counseling
(800) 452-4800

Division of Aging and
Home Services
402 W. Washington St.
P.O. Box 7083
Indianapolis, IN 46207
(800) 545-7763
(317) 232-7020

IOWA
Insurance Division
Lucas State Office
Building
East 12th and Grand St.s,
6th Floor
Des Moines, IA 50319
(515) 281-5705

Insurance Counseling
(515) 281-5705

IOWA (cont.)
Department of Elder
Affairs
Jewett Building, Suite 236
914 Grand Ave.
Des Moines, IA 50309
(515) 281-5187

KANSAS
Insurance Department
420 SW 9th St.
Topeka, KS 66612
(913) 296-3071
(800) 432-2484

Insurance Counseling
(800) 432-3535

Department on Aging
150-S. Docking State
Office Building
915 SW Harrison
Topeka, KS 66612-1500
(913) 296-4986

KENTUCKY
Insurance Department
215 W. Main St.
P.O. Box 517
Frankfort, KY 40602
(502) 564-3630

KENTUCKY (cont.)
Insurance Counseling
(800) 372-2973

Div of Aging Services
Cabinet for Human
  Resources
275 E. Main St.,
  5th Fl. West
Frankfort, KY 40621
(502) 564-6930

LOUISIANA
Insurance Department
Senior Health Insurance
  Information Program
  (SHIIP)
P.O. Box 94214
Baton Rouge, LA 70804
(504) 342-5301
(800) 259-5301

Insurance Counseling
(800) 259-5301
(504) 342-5301

Governor's Office of
  Elderly Affairs
4550 N. Blvd.
P.O. Box 80374
Baton Rouge, LA 70896
(504) 925-1700

MAINE
Bureau of Insurance
Consumer Division
State House, Station 34
Augusta, ME 04333
(207) 582-8707

Insurance Counseling
(800) 750-5353

Bureau of Elder and
  Adult Services
State House, Station 11
Augusta, ME 04333
(207) 624-5335

MARYLAND
Insurance Admin.
Complaints/Investigation
  Unit—Life and Health
501 St. Paul Place
Baltimore, MD 21202
(410) 333-2793
(410) 333-2770

Insurance Counseling
(800) 243-3425

Office on Aging
301 W. Preston St.
  Room 1004
Baltimore, MD 21201
(410) 225-1102

MASSACHUSETTS
Insurance Division
Consumer Services
  Section
470 Atlantic Ave.
Boston, MA 02210-2223
(617) 521-7777

Insurance Counseling
(800) 882-2003
(617) 727-7750

Executive Office of
Elder Affairs
1 Ashburton Place, 5th Fl.
Boston, MA 02108
(800) 882-2003
(617) 727-7750

MICHIGAN
Insurance Bureau
P.O. Box 30220
Lansing, MI 48909
(517) 373-0240 (General
  Assistance)
(517) 335-1702 (Senior
  Issues)

Insurance Counseling
(517) 373-8230

MICHIGAN (cont.)
Office of Services to the
  Aging
611 W. Ottawa St.
P.O. Box 30026
Lansing, MI 48909
(517) 373-8230

MINNESOTA
Insurance Department
Department of Commerce
133 E. 7th St.
St. Paul, MN 55101-2362
(612) 296-4026

Insurance Counseling
(800) 882-6262

Board on Aging
Human Services Building
4th Fl., 444 Lafayette Rd.
St. Paul, MN 55155-3843
(612) 296-2770

MISSISSIPPI
Insurance Department
Consumer Assistance
  Division
P.O. Box 79
Jackson, MS 39205
(601) 359-3569

Insurance Counseling
(800) 948-3090

MISSISSIPPI (cont.)
Division of Aging and
   Adult Services
750 N. State St.
Jackson, MS 39202
(800) 948-3090
(601) 359-4929

MISSOURI
Insurance Department
Consumer Services
   Section
P.O. Box 690
Jefferson City, MO
   65102-0690
(800) 726-7390
(314) 751-2640

Insurance Counseling
(800) 390-3330

Division of Aging
Department of Social
   Services
615 Howerton Court
P.O. Box 1337
Jefferson City, MO
   65102-1337
(314) 751-3082

MONTANA
Insurance Department
126 N. Sanders
Mitchell Bldg, Room 270
P.O. Box 4009
Helena, MT 59601
(406) 444-2040

Insurance Counseling
(800) 332-2272

Office on Aging
48 N. Last Chance Gulch
P.O. Box 8005
Helena, MT 59620
(800) 332-2272
(406) 444-5900

NEBRASKA
Insurance Department
Terminal Building
941 "O" St., Suite 400
Lincoln, NE 68508
(402) 471-2201

Insurance Counseling
(402) 471-4506

Department on Aging
State Office Building
301 Centennial Mall S.
Lincoln, NE 68509-5044
(402) 471-2306

NEVADA
Division of Insurance
Department of Business
and Industry
1665 Hot Springs Road,
Suite 152
Carson City, NV 89710
(800) 992-0900
(702) 687-4270

Insurance Counseling
(800) 307-4444
(702) 367-1218

**Division for Aging
Services**
Department of Human
Resources
340 N. 11th St., Suite 114
Las Vegas, NV 89101
(702) 486-3545

NEW HAMPSHIRE
Insurance Department
Life and Health Division
169 Manchester St.
Concord, NH 03301
(800) 852-3416
(603) 271-2261

Insurance Counseling
(800) 852-3388
(603) 271-4642

NEW HAMPSHIRE
(cont.)
Div of Elderly Services
Dept of Health and
Human Services
State Office Park South
115 Pleasant St.
Annex Building No. 1
Concord, NH 03301
(603) 271-4680

NEW JERSEY
Insurance Department
20 W. State St.
Roebling Bldg, CN 325
Trenton, NJ 08625
(609) 292-5363

Insurance Counseling
(800) 792-8820

Division on Aging
Department of
Community Affairs
101 S. Broad St., CN 807
Trenton, NJ 08625-0807
(800) 792-8820
(609) 894-3951

NEW MEXICO
Insurance Department
P.O. Drawer 1269
Santa Fe, NM 87504
(505) 827-4500

NEW MEXICO (cont.)
Insurance Counseling
(800) 432-2080

State Agency on Aging
La Villa Rivera Building
224 E. Palace Ave.
Santa Fe, NM 87501
(800) 432-2080
(505) 827-7640

NEW YORK
Insurance Department
160 W. Broadway
New York, NY 10013
(800) 342-3736
(212) 602-0203

Insurance Counseling
(800) 333-4114
(212) 869-3850 (New
  York City area)

State Office for
  the Aging
2 Empire State Plaza
Albany, NY 12223-0001
(800) 342-9871
(518) 474-5731

NORTH CAROLINA
Insurance Department
Seniors' Health Insurance
  Information Program
  (SHIIP)
P.O. Box 26387
Raleigh, NC 27611
(800) 662-7777
  (Consumer Services)
(919) 733-0111 (SHIIP)

Insurance Counseling
(800) 443-9354

Division of Aging
693 Palmer Drive
Caller Box 29531
Raleigh, NC 27626-0531
(919) 733-3983

NORTH DAKOTA
Insurance Department
Senior Health Insurance
  Counseling
600 E. Blvd.
Bismarck, ND 58505
(800) 247-0560
(701) 328-2440

Insurance Counseling
(800) 247-0560

NORTH DAKOTA (cont.)

Aging Services Division
Department of Human
  Services
P.O. Box 7070
Bismarck, ND 58507
(800) 755-8521
(701) 328-2577

OHIO

Insurance Department
Consumer Services
  Division
2100 Stella Court
Columbus, OH 43215
(800) 686-1526
(614) 644-2673

Insurance Counseling
(800) 686-1578

Department on Aging
50 W. Broad St., 9th Fl.
Columbus, OH 43215
(800) 282-1206
(614) 466-1221

OKLAHOMA

Insurance Department
P.O. Box 53408
Oklahoma City, OK
  73152-3408
(405) 521-6628

OKLAHOMA (cont.)

Insurance Counseling
(405) 521-6628

Aging Services Division
Department of Human
  Services
312 NE 28th St.
Oklahoma City, OK
  73125
(405) 521-2327

OREGON

**Senior Health Insurance
  Benefits Assistance**
Department of Consumer
  and Business Services
470 Labor & Indust. Bldg
Salem, OR 97310
(800) 722-4134
(503) 378-4484

Insurance Counseling
(800) 722-4134

**Senior and Disabled
  Services Division**
Dept of Human Resources
500 Summer St. NE,
  2nd Fl.
Salem, OR 97310-1015
(800) 232-3020
(503) 945-5811

PENNSYLVANIA
Insurance Department
Consumer Services
  Bureau
1321 Strawberry Square
Harrisburg, PA 17120
(717) 787-2317

Insurance Counseling
(800) 783-7067
(717) 783-8970

Department of Aging
"Apprise" Health
  Insurance Counseling
  and Assistance
400 Market St.
  State Office Bldg
Harrisburg, PA 17101
(800) 783-7067

PUERTO RICO
Insurance Commissioner
P.O. Box 8330
San Juan, PR 00910-8330
(809) 722-8686

Insurance Counseling
(809) 721-5710

PUERTO RICO (cont.)
Governor's Office of
  Elderly Affairs
Gericulture Commission
Box 11398
Santurce, PR 00910
(809) 722-2429

RHODE ISLAND
Insurance Division
233 Richmond St.,
  Suite 233
Providence, RI 02903
(401) 277-2223

Insurance Counseling
(800) 322-2880

Department of Elderly
  Affairs
160 Pine St.
Providence, RI 02903
(401) 277-2858

SOUTH CAROLINA
Insurance Department
Consumer Services
  Section
P.O. Box 100105
Columbia, SC 29202
(800) 768-3467
(803) 737-6180

SOUTH CAROLINA (cont.)
Insurance Counseling
(800) 868-9095

Division on Aging
202 Arbor Lake Drive
Suite 301
Columbia, SC 29223
(803) 737-7500

SOUTH DAKOTA
Insurance Department
500 E. Capitol Ave.
Pierre, SD 57501-5070
(605) 773-3563

Insurance Counseling
(605) 773-3656

Office of Adult Services and Aging
700 Governors Drive
Pierre, SD 57501-2291
(605) 773-3656

TENNESSEE
Insurance Department
Insurance Assistance
4th Fl., 500 James
  Robertson Pkwy
Nashville, TN 37243
(800) 525-2816
(615) 741-4955

TENNESSEE (cont.)
Insurance Counseling
(800) 525-2816

Commission on Aging
Andrew Jackson Bldg,
  9th Fl.
500 Deaderick St.
Nashville, TN 37243
(615) 74-2056

TEXAS
Insurance Department
Complaints Resolution,
  MC 111-1A
333 Guadalupe St.
P.O. Box 149091
Austin, TX 78714-9091
(800) 252-3439
(512) 463-6500

Insurance Counseling
(800) 252-3439

Department on Aging
1949 IH 35 South
P.O. Box 12786 (78711)
Austin, TX 78741
(800) 252-9240
(512) 444-2727

UTAH
Insurance Department
Consumer Services
3110 State Office Bldg
Salt Lake City, UT
  84114-6901
(800) 429-3805
(801) 538-3805

Insurance Counseling
(800) 606-0608
(801) 538-3910

Division of Aging and
  Adult Services
120 North 200 West
Salt Lake City, UT 84103
(800) 606-0608

VERMONT
Dept of Banking
  and Insurance
Consumer Complaint Div
89 Main St., Drawer 20
Montpelier, VT
  05620-3101
(802) 828-3302

Insurance Counseling
(800) 828-3302

VERMONT (cont.)
Department of Aging
  and Disabilities
Waterbury Complex
103 S. Main St.
Waterbury, VT 05671
(802) 241-2400

VIRGINIA
Bureau of Insurance
Consumer Services
  Division
1300 E. Main St.
P.O. Box 1157
Richmond, VA 23209
(800) 552-7945
(804) 371-9741

Insurance Counseling
(800) 552-4464

Department for Aging
700 Centre, 10th Fl.
700 E. Franklin St.
Richmond, VA 23219
(800) 552-4464
(804) 225-2271

VIRGIN ISLANDS
Insurance Department
Kongens Gade No. 18
St. Thomas, VI 00802
(809) 774-2991

VIRGIN ISLANDS
(cont.)
Insurance Counseling
(809) 774-2991

**Senior Citizen Affairs
  Division**
Dept of Human Services
19 Estate Diamond
Fredericksted
St. Croix, VI 00840
(809) 772-0930

WASHINGTON
Insurance Department
4224 6th Ave. SE, Bldg 4
P.O. Box 40256
Lacey, WA 98504-0256
(800) 562-6900
(360) 753-7300

Insurance Counseling
(800) 397-4422

**Aging and Adult
  Services Admin.**
Social and Health
  Services Department
P.O. Box 45050
Olympia, WA 98504
(360) 586-3768

WEST VIRGINIA
Insurance Department
Consumer Service Div.
2019 Washington St., E
P.O. Box 50540
Charleston, WV
  25305-0540
(800) 642-9004
(800) 435-7381 (TDD)
(304) 558-3386

Insurance Counseling
(304) 558-3317

Commission on Aging
State Capitol Complex
  Holly Grove
1900 Hanawha Blvd., E.
Charleston, WV
  25305-0160
(304) 558-3317

WISCONSIN
Insurance Department
Complaints Division
P.O. Box 7873
Madison, WI 53707
(800) 236-8517
(608) 266-0103

Insurance Counseling
(800) 242-1060

WISCONSIN (cont.)
Board on Aging and
 Long-Term Care
214 N. Hamilton St.
Madison, WI 53703
(800) 242-1060
(608) 266-8944

WYOMING
Insurance Department
Herschler Building
122 W. 25th St.
Cheyenne, WY 82002
(800) 438-5768
(307) 777-7401

Insurance Counseling
(800) 438-5768

Division on Aging
Hathaway Building
2300 Capitol Ave.,
 Room 139
Cheyenne, WY 82002
(800) 442-2766
(307) 777-7986

BIBLIOGRAPHY

Commager, Henry Steele and Nevins, Allan. 1981. *A Pocket History of the United States*. New York: Washington Square Press Publication of Pocket Books, a division of Simon and Schuster, Inc.

Commerce Clearing House. 1996. *Medicare Explained*. Chicago: Commerce Clearing House.

Commerce Clearing House. 1996. *Social Security Explained*. Chicago: Commerce Clearing House.

Department of Health and Human Services (DHHS). 1994. *Medicare and Managed Care Plans*. Publication #HCFA 02195. Washington, D.C.: U.S. Government Printing Office.

DHHS. 1994. *Medicare Pays for Flu Shots*. Publication #HCFA-10963. Washington, D.C.: U.S. Government Printing Office.

DHHS. 1994. *Consumer Fraud Pamphlet: How to Help Stop Medicare from Being Ripped-Off*. Washington, D.C.: U.S. Government Printing Office.

DHHS. 1994. *Medicare and Other Health Benefits*. Publication #HCFA 02179. Washington, D.C.: U.S. Government Printing Office.

DHHS, Bureau of Data Management and Strategy, Office of Statistics and Data Management. 1994. *1994 HCFA Statistics*. Washington, D.C.: U.S. Government Printing Office.

Health Care Financing Administration (HCFA). 1994. *1994 Data Compendium*. Washington, D.C.: U.S. Government Printing Office.

HCFA. 1995. *1995 Guide to Health Insurance for People With Medicare*. Publication #HCFA-02110. Washington, D.C.: U.S. Government Printing Office.

HCFA. 1993. *Medicare Q&A: 85 Commonly Asked Questions*. Publication #HCFA-02172. Washington, D.C.: U.S. Government Printing Office.

HCFA. 1995. *Your Medicare Handbook*. Washington, D.C.: U.S. Government Printing Office.

Knaus, Denise L. 1995. *Medicare Rules and Regulations 1995-96*. California: PMIC.

Knaus, Denise L., ed. 1991. *Payment & Postpayment Procedures and Disclosure of Information*. Vol. 6 of *Medicare Rules and Regulations*. New York: McGraw-Hill.

Knaus, Denise L., ed. 1991. *Reasonable Charges*. Vol. 3 of *Medicare Rules and Regulations*. New York: McGraw-Hill.

Legal Counsel for the Elderly. 1991. *Medicare Practice Manual*. Washington, D.C.: American Association of Retired Persons.

Social Security Administration. 1995. Interview by author. Downers Grove, Illinois, 11/95.

Blue Shield of California. 1995. Materials and lectures at the Medifest '95 conference, 26-29 July, at Hyatt Embarcadero, San Francisco, CA.

INDEX